HUMAN AND ETHICAL ISSUES
IN THE SURGICAL CARE OF PATIENTS
WITH LIFE-THREATENING DISEASE

HUMAN AND ETHICAL ISSUES IN THE SURGICAL CARE OF PATIENTS WITH LIFE-THREATENING DISEASE

THE BRITISH SCHOOL OF OSTEOPATHY,
1-4 SUFFOLK ST., LONDON. SW1Y 4HG
TEL. 01 - 930 9254-8

Edited By

FREDERIC P. HERTER

KENNETH FORDE

LESTER C. MARK

ROBERT DeBELLIS

AUSTIN H. KUTSCHER

FLORENCE SELDER

With the Editorial Assistance of

LILLIAN G. KUTSCHER

A FOUNDATION OF THANATOLOGY TEXT

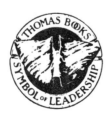

CHARLES C THOMAS • PUBLISHER
Springfield • Illinois • U.S.A.

Published and Distributed Throughout the World by

CHARLES C THOMAS • PUBLISHER
2600 South First Street
Springfield, Illinois 62717

This book is protected by copyright. No part of it
may be reproduced in any manner without written
permission from the publisher.

© *1986 by* CHARLES C THOMAS • PUBLISHER

ISBN 0-398-05194-1

Library of Congress Catalog Card Number: 85-20120

With **THOMAS BOOKS** *careful attention is given to all details of manufacturing and design. It is the Publisher's desire to present books that are satisfactory as to their physical qualities and artistic possibilities and appropriate for their particular use.* THOMAS BOOKS *will be true to those laws of quality that assure a good name and good will.*

Printed in the United States of America
SC-R-3

Library of Congress Cataloging-in-Publication Data
Main entry under title:

Human and ethical issues in the surgical care of
patients with life-threatening disease.

"A Foundation of Thanatology Text."
Includes bibliographies and index.
1. Critically ill—Surgery—Moral and ethical
aspects. 2. Terminally ill—Surgery—Moral and ethical
aspects. 3. Critically ill—Surgery—Psychological
aspects. 4. Terminally ill—Surgery—Psychological
aspects. 5. Surgery—Decision making. 6. Death—
Psychological aspects. I. Herter, Frederic P.
[DNLM: 1. Critical Care—psychology. 2. Death.
3. Ethics, Medical. 4. Surgery, Operative—psychology.
5. Terminal Care—psychology. W 50 H917]
RD27.7.H86   1986   174'.2   85-20120
ISBN 0-398-05194-1

CONTRIBUTORS

Frederic P. Herter, M.D., Auchincloss Professor of Surgery, College of Physicians and Surgeons, Columbia University, New York, New York

Kenneth Forde, M.D., Professor of Clinical Surgery, College of Physicians and Surgery, Columbia University, New York, New York

Lester C. Mark, M.D., Professor of Anesthesiology, College of Physicians and Surgeons, Columbia University, New York, New York

Robert DeBellis, M.D., Assistant Professor of Clinical Medicine, College of Physicians and Surgeons, Columbia University, New York, New York

Austin H. Kutscher, D.D.S., Professor of Dentistry (in Psychiatry), Department of Psychiatry, College of Physicians and Surgeons, Columbia University; Professor of Dentistry (in Psychiatry), Division of Oral and Maxillofacial Surgery, School of Dental and Oral Surgery, Columbia University, New York, New York; President, The Foundation of Thanatology

Florence Selder, Ph.D., Associate Professor and Urban Research Center Scientist, University of Wisconsin, Milwaukee, Wisconsin

****

Henry Aranow, M.D., Lambert Professor Emeritus of Medicine, College of Physicians and Surgeons, Columbia University, New York, New York

Jean M. Barsa, M.D., Department of Radiation Medicine, St. Vincent's Hospital and Medical Center, New York, New York

Henrik H. Bendixen, M.D., Professor and Chairman, Department of Anesthesiology, College of Physicians and Surgeons, Columbia University, New York, New York

Robert G. Bertsch, M.D., Associate Professor of Surgery, College of Physicians and Surgeons, Columbia University, New York, New York

Richard S. Blacher, M.D., Clinical Professor of Psychiatry and Lecturer in Surgery, Tufts New England Medical Center, Boston, Massachusetts

Eliabeth J. Clark, Ph.D., A.C.S.W., Department of Health Professions, Montclair State College, Upper Montclair, New Jersey

John Conley, M.D., Professor Emeritus of Clinical Otolaryngology, College of Physicians and Surgeons, Columbia University, New York, New York

Frederick A. Ehlert, Class of 1986, College of Physicians and Surgeons, Columbia University, New York, New York

Eli Ginzberg, Ph.D., Director, Conservation of Human Resources, Columbia College, New York, New York

Frederick M. Golomb, M.D., Professor of Clinical Surgery, New York University Medical Center, New York, New York

David V. Habif, M.D., Morris and Rose Milstein Professor of Surgery, College of Physicians and Surgeons, Columbia University, New York, New York

Mahlon S. Hale, M.D., Associate Professor of Psychiatry, University of Connecticut Health Center, Farmington, Connecticut

Father Jefferson J. Hammer, Director of Pastoral Care, St. Vincent's Hospital and Medical Center, New York, New York

Milton W. Hamolsky, M.D., Professor of Medical Science and Co-Chairman, Section of Medicine, Brown University School of Medicine; Physician-in-Chief and Chairman, Department of Medicine, Rhode Island Hospital, Providence, Rhode Island

Allen I. Hyman, M.D., Associate Professor of Anesthesiology and Pediatrics, College of Physicians and Surgeons, Columbia University, New York, New York

Alfred Jaretzki, III, M.D., Associate Professor of Clinical Surgery, College of Physicians and Surgeons, Columbia University, New York, New York

Thomas C. King, M.D., Jose M. Ferrer, Jr. Professor of Surgery, College of Physicians and Surgeons, Columbia University, New York, New York

Lillian G. Kutscher, Publications Editor, The Foundation of Thanatology, New York, New York

Phyllis C. Leppert, M.D., Assistant Professor of Obstetrics and Gynecology, College of Physicians and Surgeons, Columbia University, New York, New York

Paul LoGerfo, M.D., Associate Professor of Surgery and Director of Surgical Oncology, College of Physicians and Surgeons, Columbia University, New York, New York

Abraham Lurie, Ph.D., Director, Department of Social Work Services, Long Island Jewish-Hillside Medical Center, New Hyde Park, New York

Russell Lynes, Writer and Patient, New York, New York

Mary McGrath, M.D., Assistant Professor of Surgery, Division of Plastic and Reconstructive Surgery, College of Physicians and Surgeons, Columbia University, New York, New York

Jay I. Meltzer, M.D., Clinical Professor of Medicine, College of Physicians and Surgeons, Columbia University, New York, New York

The Right Reverend Paul Moore, Jr., The Bishop of New York, Cathedral of St. John the Divine, New York, New York

Karin M. Muraszko, M.D., Resident in Neurosurgery, College of Physicians and Surgeons, Columbia University, New York, New York

Harris M. Nagler, M.D., Assistant Professor of Urology, College of Physicians and Surgeons, Columbia University, New York, New York

Vanderlyn R. Pine, Ph.D., Professor of Sociology, State University of New York at New Paltz, New York

Elizabeth Rand, M.D., Department of Psychiatry, University of Connecticut Health Center, Farmington, Connecticut

Keith Reemtsma, M.D., Valentine Mott and Johnson and Johnson Professor of Surgery; Chairman, Department of Surgery, College of Physicians and Surgeons, Columbia University, New York, New York

Harold M. Schoolman, M.D., Clinical Professor of Medicine, Georgetown University School of Medicine, Washington, D.C.; formerly, Acting Director, National Library of Medicine, National Institutes of Health, Department of Health and Human Services, Washington, D.C.

Henry M. Spotnitz, M.D., Associate Professor of Surgery, College of Physicians and Surgeons, Columbia University, New York, New York

Laurie A. Stevens, M.D., Instructor in Psychiatry, College of Physicians and Surgeons, Columbia University, New York, New York

Constance Weiskopf, R.N., M.S.N., Department of Psychiatry, University of Connecticut Health Center, Farmington, Connecticut

FOREWORD

FREDERIC P. HERTER

The problems to be explored in this volume are not directed to surgeons alone, nor simply to patients facing surgical treatment. They apply to *all* persons involved in critical illness, be they on the giving or the receiving end. Thus there are contributions from representatives of many disciplines; in addition to surgeons of varied specialty interests, there are medical oncologists, psychiatrists, members of the clergy, nurses, social workers, medical students, even patients—the whole gamut of individuals who singly or jointly bear some responsibility for the awesome transition from health to grave disease, and, ultimately, from life to death. It is that transition which will be probed.

Much has been written about cancer as the prototypical life-threatening disease, and we shall inevitably use it as a model in these discussions. But we are, in fact, speaking of all forms of critical illness that carry the immediate, or deferred threat of death. If emphasis appears to be centered on cancer, it is only that this model lends itself to a structured analysis—it has a recognizable beginning, definable stages in its progress, and, in its worst expression, an inexorable ending. Each phase of the disease, starting with the initial diagnosis, and proceeding through the prognostic implications determined by the pathology to the dreaded appearance of metastases and the recognition of incurability, has its own characteristic impact on patient and physician alike. These sequential "crises" are readily identifiable in cancer, but they can be found in a variety of irreversible disorders of differing origin. The nature of the disease is irrelevant; what *is* important that at each stage in the evolution of the illness, from its inception to its terminal finality, the patient is faced not only with a new set of threatening circumstances but with an ever changing support system. The initial pivotal role of the surgeon, established during the diagnosis and primary treatment of the disease, may be transferred to others as the illness progresses and as new forms of therapy become necessary. For a short while the radiotherapist may assume the mantle of care. Chemotherapy may then be indicated, and again the prime responsibility for patient care is transferred, this time to an oncologist. When all therapies are found to be fruitless in the face of advancing disease, the main support system may revert to the local physician, or to an unintegrated team of nurses, clergy, psychiatrists, and social service workers.

All too often the dying patient becomes lost or neglected as the scene changes and a new cast of characters is introduced. No one seems to be directing the show, and unless family support is strong, the patient feels abandoned at a time when concern and care are most needed. Of all the recognized forms of suffering, this can be the most tragic.

There are no easy answers to this dilemma, nor stock solutions that apply in all instances. What is vital to the patient is that transfers in responsibility for care be orderly and fully understood, and that decisions regarding change be arrived at by doctor and patient together. The surgeon, so central in importance to the patient during the early and hopeful stages of the disease, should relinquish his responsibilities *only* if other key figures in the care system can be identified and agreed upon. These might include the family physician who made the original referral, or the oncologist who conducts the chemotherapy over a protracted period of time, or a strong and close member of the family, or one of the clergy—or, if none of the above is accessible or willing, the surgeon himself, though he is dealing with disciplines far removed from surgery. But someone must be there to orchestrate care, and to hold the hand.

Other issues are dealt with in equal depth in this compendium, and they are presented in some sequential order. Opening chapters deal with the preparation of the patient for surgery. Commonly held fears about surgery, both real and imagined, are explored, as well as the importance of patient attitudes in confronting possibly life-threatening procedures or conditions. The dehumanizing hospital environment, particularly as related to intensive care, is given due attention, as well as the threat to sexuality and body function and control imposed by the surgery itself. The focus then moves on to the progression of the disease process and the expansion or sharing of the care base, necessitating the shifts in responsibility alluded to above. The particular role of each discipline in this "team" effort is described. Lastly, there is discussion of the terminal phases of the disease, that final transition from life to death in which the concern and skills of all components of the care system are so severely challenged. The choice of institutional, hospice or home care is debated, as well as the various approaches to the relief of suffering, be it physical, emotional or spiritual, evinced by the dying patient.

No treatise on critical illness can be complete without some mention of the many ethical dilemmas which face the responsible members of the care team. When should aggressive therapy be discontinued for the ostensibly incurable patient, to be replaced by simple measures designed for comfort only? How should the limited resources of a hospital, in terms of specialty or intensive care, be allocated? Should age, or disease type, or economic resources, enter these decisions? How, and for how long, should artificial life-sustaining devices be employed? How are differences in opinion between the professional staff and the patient's family reconciled? What is informed consent? Are candor and truth synonymous? Is clinical research antithetical to the patient's interests?

These are a few of the troublesome questions which are addressed, if not completely answered, in this volume.

The last group of papers relate to education. It was not long ago that issues pertaining to death and dying were absent from medical school curricula. There is now a voluminous literature on the subject. "Thanatology" has become more than an abstraction, and the last twenty years has seen a minor revolution in the thinking and education of all health-care practitioners. More, obviously, has to be done. Although the level of consciousness with respect to death-related issues has risen, thanatology is far from being a science, and we are only marginally better in dealing with the critically ill or dying patient.

But discussions such as these, subjective or theoretical as they may be, are useful. It is futile to believe that there are absolute answers to many of the questions raised; nor, perhaps, should there be. The wonders and mysteries of human behavior, particularly as it applies to death, will continue to defy scientific analysis. Yet in exploring these issues we are forced to put our own thoughts, emotions, prejudices in some sort of order, and in so doing perhaps help ourselves to become more understanding as persons and more effective as doctors.

ACKNOWLEDGMENT

The focus of the discipline of thanatology is on the art of enhancing humanitarian caregiving for patients who are critically, chronically, or terminally ill, with equal concern exhibited for the well-being of their family members. From a base in thanatology, interdisciplinary professionals are dedicated to promoting vastly improved psychosocial and medical care for these patients and assistance for their families. Proposed is a philosophy of caregiving that reinforces alternative ways of supporting positive qualities in the lives of those who are critically ill, life-threatened, or dying and that introduces methods of intervention on behalf of the emotional support of their family members and bereaved survivors.

The editors wish to acknowledge the support and encouragement of The Foundation of Thanatology in the preparation of this volume. All royalties from the sale of this book are assigned to The Foundation of Thanatology, a tax-exempt, not-for-profit, public, scientific, and educational foundation.

CONTENTS

HUMAN AND ETHICAL ISSUES IN THE SURGICAL CARE OF PATIENTS WITH LIFE-THREATENING DISEASE

Part I
PREPARATION OF THE PATIENT FOR SURGERY

1

THE WILL TO LIVE: DOES IT BEAR ON PROGNOSIS AND RECOVERY

Jefferson J. Hammer

I own the personal diary of a federal sailor captured during the Civil War who was interned in the infamous Confederate prison at Andersonville, Georgia. He was 32 years of age at the time of his capture in September of 1863. He was a carpenter by profession; married; the father of two young girls. His name—Frederick Augustus James.

James was a man energetically dedicated to the task of surmounting the hazards of prison. To achieve this, *he read:* "We have been fortunate enough to obtain the loan of quite a number of readable books from the citizen prisoners"; *he wrote:* "I wrote to my wife September 22nd and every fortnight thereafter"; *he sold:* "Sold some of my Harpers magazines, .50 and .75 each"; *he exercised:* "I find that more exercise outdoors is essential to my health"; *he cooked* his meals: "Baked a couple of corn cakes in the morning and had some boiled rice for supper"; and he began each entry of his diary with the positive statement: "a pleasant day."

He became ill in August of 1864 of what was later determined to be dysentery and diarrhea. His last entry, on August 27, 1864, reads: "Wore a wet girdle around my waist last night and so have slept much better than some days before." James died September 15, 1864.

He was a man faced with the very real possibility of dying in confinement—away from home, with strangers, prematurely, with unfulfilled responsibilities toward wife and children. It was not an accepted finality for this man and so he looked for alternate routes to survive, to

5

live. He did not agree to all means to save his life. Violence and escape were not among his options. Prisoners were being shot at Andersonville, escape tunnels discovered and their users punished severely; northern lines were hundreds of miles away.

James carefully analyzed his situation, determined his goals and resources, selected some means as possible of achievement and rejected others as unacceptable. Motivated by a clear and strong will to live, he came close to success.

It is not certain why his driving forces were insufficient to save him. The documentation of 13,000 other men dying in the same horror demonstrates that James was not a weak man unto himself. He was truly a person with a wish to survive, with a will to live.

The science of medicine has done much over the years to identify the various and complex and interacting systems of the human body but two systems need more emphasis: (1) the healing system by which the body mobilizes all its resources to combat disease; and (2) the faith (or belief) system which represents the extremely unique property of human beings that makes it possible for the human mind to affect the working of the body. The two systems—healing and faith—work together. How one responds—emotionally, intellectually, spiritually—to personal problems has a great deal to do with the way the body functions, combats disease, and recovers. The faith system is not just a state of mind; it is a prime physiological reality.

The human healing system has been shaped over millions of years of evolution to cope not merely with disorder but with detours and deflections. The process of selecting alternate routes in the face of obstacles to one's chosen goals aids not merely in achieving some secondary goal, it also strengthens and enhances the human character because a goal is reached, failure avoided, and life made better. One of the physician's main functions is to encourage, and to engage to the fullest, the patient's own ability to recognize, mobilize, and activate the forces of mind and body in turning back disease.

The art—not the science—of the doctor is to convey the possibilities of the human healing system to individuals who are conditioned to thinking of illness mainly in terms of pain, suspicious growths, surgery, prescriptions, hospital beds, and personnel. This is one reason why medical education should—must—produce men and women who are not just well trained in the science of the human body but educated as well in the human personality.

The patient's belief in the healing power of the physician is often more important than the treatment itself in reversing the course of the illness. The physician must supply not just scientific competence but also the spiritual nourishment that his patient so dearly requires. The most potent medicine available to the physician is the confidence placed in him by the patient.

Patients tend to move in the direction of their hopes or their fears. If they have strong confidence in themselves and in their physicians, they tend to have a better outcome than if they are morose and defeatist. Those patients who have a fighting spirit and who are not willing to accept a negative verdict are far more likely to improve than those who respond with a stoic acceptance of feelings colored by hopelessness and helplessness. It makes no sense to believe that only negative emotions have an effect on the body chemistry. Every emotion, negative or positive, makes its registration on the body's systems.

The human body experiences a tremendous gravitational pull in the direction of hope. That is why the patient's hopes are the physician's secret weapon. They are the hidden ingredient in any prescription. The physician is most wise to elicit everything he can to bolster attitudes, nourish the patient's outlook on life, and encourage confidence in the patient. It is essential never to underestimate the capacity of the human mind and body to regenerate—even when prospects appear the poorest.

The fact that cancer is an extreme form of human illness does not mean that all established principles for combating disease cease to have validity. One of those principles holds that even as disease is attacked, the patient must be supported in every way. Indeed, the more radical the treatment, the more important it becomes to fortify and put to work the individual's own resources—a healthy life style, a robust will to live, a meaningful support system of family and of friends, a determination to make the most out of whatever is possible. These are intangibles, to be sure, but intangibles define the human being. Love is an intangible, but no less real than the pulsating heart.

The will to live is a window on the future. It opens the individual to such help as the outside world has to offer and it connects that help to the body's own capacity to fight disease. It enables the human body and the human person to make the most of itself. The unbearable tragedy is not death—far from that—it is dying in an alien environment, separated from dignity, separated from the warmth of familiar things, separated from the ever-desired ministrations of a loving relationship of family, friends, and physician. The doctor's respect for life—even in the worst of circumstances—this is the vital ingredient of his art.

People who are seriously ill need to believe that they have a chance for recovery. They respond not only to the doctor's attitude but also to the mood of the people very close to them. If hope is missing in the eyes and the voices of their families, the absence will be felt. And so, if only in terms of the ricochet effect on patients, doctors must extend their art of healing and believing to the entire network of family and friends.

The treatment of the patient is incomplete if it is confined to diagnosis and the administration of medicines and surgical procedures. It becomes complete only when the patient's own resources and capacities are engaged. This is where the science of medicine and the art of medicine come together. What is the most painful and devastating question that can be raised about medical practice today? It is not whether physicians are up to date in their knowledge and their techniques but whether too many of them know more about illness than about the person in whom the illness exists.

One of the greatest needs in contemporary medical education is to attract students who are well rounded human beings themselves; who will be interested in people and not just in the diseases that affect them; who can comprehend the reality of suffering and not just its symptoms; whose prescription pads will not exclude the human touch and who will take into account not merely malevolent microorganisms but all the forces that exercise a downward pull on the health of patients.

It has been suggested that there exists a very high correlation between positive response to surgery and other modes of treatment, and positive attitudes by the patient both to the disease and to life in a more general sense. There exist three extremely important and interacting factors that need to be recognized and brought to light: the belief system of the patient; the belief system of the family and of those who surround the patient and who are meaningful to the patient; and the belief system of the physician himself. These positive belief systems that support and strengthen the will to live of the patient, family, and physician must be based on as valid a foundation of circumstances as possible.

There is one serious caution in this discussion, namely, the will to live is a conditioned one and great sensitivity must be exercised toward those who have clearly and objectively determined that "a fullness of life" has been achieved and thus possess a selfless lack of motivation to continue. The incentive to live must be one in which the patient inwardly and totally believes. It is not the "everything to live for" in the eyes of the world that keeps one alive but the "something" which meets the individual's own uncompromising measure of what is worth living for.

It is certain that men do reach the predetermined goals of life and having achieved the utmost—with no expectation to surpass self—conclude that there is nothing more for them to do. There are times when a person reaches a sense of weariness. People have the right to withdraw from a struggle that has no satisfactory outcome. When the longing for peace outweighs the joy of struggle for achievement, when the determination to seek peace becomes irreversible and conclusive, then the person dies. Goals satisfied, children raised, obligations fulfilled, expectations realized—these and many other things—give peace to a man and remove from him the drive to live and the fear of dying.

It is possible that the motivations and anxieties of relatives, friends, even physician, strive to override the acceptance of the patient to the proximate circumstance of the termination of life. Phrases of concern as "you have so much to live for," "I can't live without you," "what will happen to us"—can harm the patient who has achieved the finality of his life. The wife who challenges her husband to surrender his complacent state of mind and will; the doctor who offers expectations beyond realistic parameters because he has "to do something" for the patient of many years' association; the young physician who has "one more" procedure to try, all can do so much to undermine and destroy the homeostasis, the balance, of the patient well prepared to die.

A highly developed purpose and the will to live are among the prime raw materials of human existence; purpose and will may well represent the most potent forces within human reach. All persons must accept a certain measure of responsibility for their own recovery from disease and disability. Homeostatic response is the natural process that enables the organism to return to the normal state in which it was before receiving a threatening disturbance from a noxious influence. The mechanisms of the healing power of the body are so effective that many diseases are self-terminating. Good medical care does, of course, make the healing more complete, more rapid and more comfortable but in the final analysis, recovery depends upon the mobilization of the patient's own mechanisms of resistance to disease.

The will to live is not a theoretical abstraction but a physiological reality with therapeutic characteristics. The highest task of the doctor is, perhaps, to encourage to the fullest the patient's will to live and to mobilize the natural resources of the body and mind to combat disease. We should never underestimate the capacity of the human mind to regenerate, even when the prospects appear the most wretched. Protecting and cherishing the natural drives toward perfectibility and regeneration may well represent the finest exercise of human freedom.

2

PATIENTS' FEARS: REALISTIC AND UNREALISTIC

RICHARD S. BLACHER

"When they take my heart out to put it on the machine, will my heart be in the same room as my body?" This startling question, recently asked by a well-educated professional person who is contemplating coronary surgery the next day, indicated that the patient knew very little about the operative procedure. This was so, despite the fact that a careful explanation of the operation had been given to him during the previous week.

Physicians have the naive idea that patients can understand what happens to them in illness and surgery. We make the natural error of believing that if *we* know and decide something, our listeners will understand and know what we are talking about. I would offer that this is most unrealistic.

Why should patients have such a difficulty in understanding the illness and treatment? The multiple reasons for this difference in what we know and do and what patients *think* we know and do will be addressed here.

For the physician, illness may be a bacteriological, physiological, biochemical, histological, or pathological phenomenon. For the patient, illness is a mysterious, even magical event and often one of the most important events in his life. Nowhere is this more striking than in a surgical situation.

A series of difficulties prevents patients from understanding their own illness, and these include communication of medical knowledge, the hierarchy of importance of organs, personal history, social factors, and universal and idiosyncratic fantasies.

11

COMMUNICATION OF MEDICAL INFORMATION

Physicians often assume that an educated layperson shares with the physician the corpus of medical knowledge which the latter uses in everyday practice. In reality, this is not so. For example: Patients undergoing herniorrhaphy may worry unduly about the loss of testes in the surgery, since examination for the condition takes place in the genital region. Beyond this, the actual details of a hernia are quite unknown to most laymen. In a study on patients' reactions in the recovery room (Winkelstein, Blacher, and Meyer n.d.), we sought a group of patients who, while awake, had surgery for a benign condition. We selected a group of patients who had had herniorrhaphy under spinal anesthesia. To our surprise, when we introduced ourselves, the first question most patients asked was, "What did they find?" We certainly had not anticipated that these patients would worry about malignancy and yet the question obviously indicated such a concern.

KNOWLEDGE

Because of a lack of knowledge the words of the physician may be taken quite literally at times.

> A successful, 50-year-old business executive was seen nine years following successful coronary artery surgery, because he found himself increasingly anxious. Although he was in excellent health he had recently quit his job, a job that gave him much satisfaction. When asked about this job change he noted that he had only a year to live—as a matter of fact a year and a month. This decision piqued the interviewer's curiosity and further questioning revealed that before surgery he was told that his condition was such that he might die in a month; after the surgery his surgeon had, in passing, mentioned that the surgery would add 10 years to his life. This meant to him that he had 10 years and 1 month to live and now that the 9 years were up he thought that he would get his affairs in order and prepare for the end.

Another problem of language has especially to do with those words that have technical meanings in medicine and different meanings in the lay vocabulary. Nowhere is this more striking than in cardiology. Patients, who are told that they have heart failure, assume this to be a terminal diagnosis. Heart block, rather than an EKG finding, is taken to mean that something is obstructing the blood flow to the heart. Such terms are common in medicine, and it is easy for the patient to misinterpret the meaning of the physician.

ORGAN HIERARCHY

There is no question that most patients have their own hierarchy of organ importance. For example, in discussing his impending valve replacement, an anxious man noted that his nervousness was because he felt that his heart was a vital organ. The interviewer, playing devil's advocate, suggested that other organs were vital also. The patient smiled and said, "Yes, but the heart is the *most* vital."

The brain is high on patients' lists, as are the kidneys and gastrointestinal tract. The pancreas, and in this country, the liver, may be thought of as silent organs, without much of a psychic representation in most patients. If given the choice, it would not surprise us if patients chose pancreatectomy over circumcision, despite the reality of the situation to the physician. It may be unreasonable for the doctor to expect patients to understand the importance of all their organs.

PERSONAL HISTORY

Since we are all children of our own childhood, previous experiences naturally inform the present, and the earlier we are exposed to traumatic episodes, the more influential they may be in our later development. We may see this in all manner of ways in hospitalized patients, and sometimes these effects of early experiences may be striking. We have seen patients who have developed a great deal of anxiety immediately on admission to the hospital for whatever surgery they were to undergo. From some of these patients we have learned that they have had an early hospitalization and surgery. Those experiences combined the pain of the procedure and the separation from home. At times, connecting the current anxiety and the early experience may be very salutary for the patient as he sees that his anxiety is not due to current medical situations but rather to the dreaded anticipations of earlier years.

Another example of past history affecting the present is seen in postoperative depressions. In our experience, the most common cause of this condition is a variant of survivor guilt. The majority of patients who are depressed after surgery give a history of close members of the family who have died at an age younger than theirs, either from the same illness for which the patient has had successful surgery or from a condition that patients consider less serious than theirs. This is a paradoxical reaction since quite often, in a serious procedure such as cardiac surgery, the patient did not expect to survive. The reason for this condition is found in the "quantitative" view of life that many people have. It is felt that nature demands a certain percentage of fatalities, and therefore if another person dies, then one's chances of surviving are enhanced. It becomes then a situation where the patient feels that parents' or siblings' death has allowed him, the patient, to live. The theme is "as long as one of us has to die, I am glad it wasn't I." On another level, of course, this means "I am glad he died" and the patient is not able to tolerate this without an enormous sense of guilt. Thus, he becomes depressed.

FANTASIES

Every surgical intervention is both an anxiety provoking exploration and a dangerous situation in which one might be mutilated or changed in some way. The term "minor surgery" must be considered a surgical term since it is rare that a patient reacts to even the most benign procedure with equanimity. Any surgery is only minor in comparison with other surgery. It is not uncommon for our patients confronting heart surgery to note that their previous surgeries had all been minor—thus cholecystectomies, hip replacements, and colonic resections may be described as "nothing major" when the patient is asked about prior operations.

Some fantasies are shared by many if not most patients undergoing certain procedures. For example, patients who anticipate heart surgery have the universal statistic, despite what they may have been told by the surgeon, that the risk for death is 50-50. This figure seems to represent not only the danger of having one's heart operated upon but, as well, represents the unique way that the heart functions. It is either on, in which case one lives, or it is off and one dies.

Another fantasy shared by many cardiac patients is that while they are on bypass and their heart is not functioning they are dead. Since it is the historical basis for defining life and death, the heart beat is still used in this way. Despite the fact that current medical knowledge indicates that the status of the brain is the landmark for the definition of death, the heart is still viewed by both laymen and many medical people as the organ of importance. [I have discussed elsewhere (Blacher 1983) the implications that this fantasy of death and resurrection might have on contemplating the surgery.] Most cardiac patients are quite calm before surgery, but an occasional patient is quite anxious. That patient often is a devout believer in an afterlife. His fantasy usually is, that during the surgery and while on bypass he will be dead and his soul will go to heaven. There he will see close members of the family—often parents who have died when the patient was quite young—and then be in conflict. When the surgeon starts his heart surgery, should he stay in heaven with his parents or should he return to his family on earth? This is dealt with by the patient quite in geographic terms and it is not experienced as some theoretical construct.

While there may be universal fantasies, most patients have to struggle with their own personal views of body function. One such patient approached the surgeon with a request that while his valve was being removed that the bitterness be removed from his heart. This patient was indeed an embittered person, but when I asked him about this thought he made it quite clear that this was not a metaphorical statement. Did he really think that his bitter feeling came from something in his heart? "Where else would it come from?" he replied.

As transplant procedures become more common the fantasy of the patients that they acquire characteristics from the donor will probably increase. This thought is common enough in its context. In the early days of blood transfusion, when patients lay side by side, it did not seem strange to the recipient to have thoughts of having taken part of the other person within him. One such man described that for months after the procedure he walked around using an Irish brogue in imitation of the donor. Basch (1973) has pointed to such reactions in kidney transplant patients. One example was a young man who learned that his donor had certain traits that he detested. He thereupon stopped taking his anti-rejection medication and died.

Practical Effects

In themselves, these fantasies are of interest to our understanding of the patient. Beyond this, and from the surgical point of view, obviously more important is the fact that they influence the patient's behavior in many ways. For example, patients may refuse to have important procedures because their anticipations are different from the surgeons. One such patient, a highly intelligent professional person, opted against a much needed herniorrhaphy until he revealed that his decision was based on his anticipation that of course he would lose his testes in the process. A simple explanation clarified the issue and he signed permission. I have seen patients who have been unable to accept heart surgery until the fantasy that they would be dead and visiting their family members in heaven had been clarified and discussed. For some of them a simple statement that they will *not* be dead during the procedure can be very reassuring.

Sometimes the patient's view of reality may seem more frightening than reality itself. In discussing how patients viewed their valve surgery I have had numbers of patients say, "They take your heart and lungs out and put them on the machine." We listeners would be quite upset at hearing such a statement. When asked, then, how they replaced the valve the patient would stammer and say something to the effect of "Oh, they have ways—they use instruments and wires." When finally asked if they had to open the heart to replace the valve, the patient would blanch and vigorously deny this possibility despite his willingness to have his heart removed. All of these patients had had careful explanations of the procedure using a model of the heart to demonstrate the replacement. Despite this three-dimensional explanation, most of the patients queried (Blacher 1971) insisted that their hearts had not been opened. The implications for conformed consent are quite clear in this and, of course, are of great concern to surgeons. A study by Robinson and Merav (1976) demonstrated the great difficulty cardiac patients had in recalling what had transpired at their interview with the surgeon. Interviews were tape recorded and when the other surgeon queried the patient 4 to 6 months later most of the major issues discussed were forgotten. Sixteen of the twenty patients insisted that certain important topics had never been discussed. Although the interviews lasted over 20 minutes, several of the patients complained that they were told nothing. "All he did was lift up my shirt, put a stethoscope on my heart and that was it." They also noted that those patients who could recall least were most authoritative in stating their recollections, false as these recollections were.

What the surgeon does and what the patient thinks he does are not only often different because of the patient's lack of surgical knowledge, they are often different because what the patient can tolerate may be far different from what his medical attendants think he can. It behooves us to remember that the patient's view of reality is for him much more important than what actually occurs in the operating theatre.

REFERENCES

Basch, S.H. 1973. "The Intrapsychic Integration of a New Organ." *Psychoanalytic Quarterly* 42:364–384.

Blacher, R.S. 1971. "Open-Heart Surgery—The Patient's Point of View." *The Mount Sinai Journal of Medicine* 38:74–78.

Blacher, R.S. 1983. "Death, Resurrection, and Rebirth: Observations in Cardiac Surgery." *Psychoanalytic Quarterly* 52:56–72.

Robinson, A. and A. Merav. 1976. "Informed Consent: Recall by Patients Tested Postoperatively." *Annals of Thoracic Surgery* 22:209–219.

Winkelstein, C., R.S. Blacher, and B.C. Meyer. 1965. Unpublished data.

3

PREPARATION OF THE PATIENT
AND FAMILY FOR MAJOR SURGERY

ALFRED JARETZKI III

INTRODUCTION

The psychological preparation of the patient for a major operation is the responsibility of the surgeon and is essential to a successful outcome. In my experience, this can best be accomplished by combining the psychological preparation unobtrusively with the patient's evaluation and preoperative management.

The goal of the psychological preparation is to develop a relationship ,between the patient and the surgeon that gives the patient confidence, trust, and hope. To achieve this, the patient must be well informed, must be cognizant of the problems associated with the decision-making process, must be aware that major decisions may have to be made intraoperatively, must be prepared for a variable outcome, and must develop a willingness to work at recovery from the physical and psychological trauma of the operation. Since all the steps taken in the psychological preparation of the patient constitute good medicine, they should be of benefit to the patient in and by themselves; and incidentally, since these steps represent good medicine, they are the best protection against malpractice suits.

The approach the surgeon uses should be varied to fit the needs of the surgical specialty, the personality of the surgeon and, of course, the individuality of the patient. As a guide, I shall describe how the initial consultation and the preoperative visit can be used to achieve these goals. Although each step plays an important role in patient evaluation,

19

my comments will be primarily confined to the part these steps play in his psychological preparation. Since consciously or unconsciously, the patient's assessment of the surgeon's intraoperative judgment and skill is based upon what the patient sees in the surgeon preoperatively, if these steps are done well, confidence and trust will be nurtured.

INITIAL CONSULTATION

The initial contact with the patient is important. A well-orchestrated interview can result in the surgeon knowing a great deal about the patient's psychological make-up and the patient developing confidence and trust in the surgeon. My recommendations for this visit are:

1. The initial contact should be in the office when possible rather than the hospital room. In this way, the patient is better able to maintain his own self image, there is less depersonalization, and the patient has more time to consider the recommendations and can do so in his own environment.

2. One or more family members, or a close friend, should be present. Since trust and confidence by members of the family can be supportive to the patient and lack of trust by them destructive, the psychological preparation of the family is also important.

3. Enough time should be allotted to give the patient undivided attention. Nothing is more damaging than to appear disinterested or give the impression of treating a disease rather than an individual.

4. The surgeon should demonstrate complete command of the previously available material and x-rays at this visit. To do otherwise consciously or unconsciously raises the fear that there are important events in the medical history that the surgeon may not know.

5. The pertinent history should be reviewed with the patient even though the details may already be recorded. It gives the surgeon the opportunity to assure himself of the accuracy of the facts, new details frequently put the problem in a different perspective, and the patient has the opportunity to be heard.

6. At the least, a limited physical exam should be performed. The advantage gained medically is obvious; the gain to the patient in the "laying on of hands" has been well documented.

7. Important verification data such as previous operative notes and

pathological slides should be requested. This information may be pertinent and should be obtained. The request itself sets the stage for a better understanding by the patient of the decision-making process.

The stage having been set by the preceding events, the next steps are critical.

8. The physician should discuss with the patient the impression and recommendations—starting with a brief review of the facts, the differential diagnoses, the most likely diagnosis, the additional studies that are needed and why—and then make a tentative recommendation including a description of the available alternatives. These maneuvers get the patient intimately involved in the decision-making process, allow the patient to see how the differential diagnosis and therapeutic recommendations have developed as a natural consequence of the available data, and allow the patient to acquire the knowledge necessary to understand the recommendations and make an informed judgment. They also give the patient the feeling of control which is important in his psychological preparation.

In discussing the differential diagnosis, it is important to begin to use the words "tumor," "growth," "malignancy," and "cancer" if they apply. The use of these words, if sensitively presented, should help to evaluate the patient's understanding and ability to deal with the diagnosis, and his illness, and opens the door for the patient to express his attitudes and fears. Often, at this point, a frank discussion of the diagnosis, possible extent of disease and prognosis commences; inappropriate fears can be allayed and a pact and understanding between the surgeon and the patient begins to develop which can be helpful in the days, weeks, months or years to come.

9. Before ending this initial visit, if an operation is definitely planned, some discussion of the surgical procedure itself is appropriate. The important points that need to be made, some directly and some indirectly, are: the patient's safety and well-being are paramount; the operation will be designed so that the patient can return to active life (if applicable); a lobe or lung (in my field) will not be removed unless the patient can function effectively without it; and he is told indirectly he has a future by describing what he will be able to do after discharge from the hospital, when he will be able to resume his normal activities, and (again in my field) by insisting that stopping smoking will help him in the years ahead.

10. And finally, I believe it is extremely helpful in many instances to send the patient, or a responsible member of his family, a copy of the formal Consultation Note. This maneuver reassures the patient that information is not being withheld from him. In addition, it eliminates confusion, gives him the opportunity to review what has been discussed, make corrections, ask questions, and thereby further helps the patient become an active participant in his care.

PREOPERATIVE VISIT

The preoperative visit the day before surgery should be devoted to a discussion of the details of the perioperative period; if practical, at least one member of the family should be present. Insofar as possible, there should be no surprises to the patient postoperatively, he should be well prepared for the pain and discomfort, he should know what tubes and equipment are planned, and his responsibilities toward getting well should be clearly understood and accepted. Toward this end, in general the more details the better. If others are to be involved in his care postoperatively, such as a respiratory therapist or an intensive care unit, individuals representing these disciplines can be very helpful to the patient if he sees them too. At the least, the staff nurses and residents or physician's assistants, if they are involved, should review this with the patient as well. At this point, the patient is frequently terrified, rather than just apprehensive, and as much reinforcement as possible is needed.

It is also appropriate to review again the indication for the procedure, what is planned, the anticipated outcome, and tell him again when it is expected that he will go home, what he will be doing as he recovers, and when he can return to his normal activities.

Before leaving the patient, I review the meaning of the informed consent by providing (asking him to read and sign, or in some instances summarizing only) a seven point addendum to the hospital consent form which I have prepared (see attached). Although the wording may seem frightening and I doubt this addendum will prove of particular benefit in a court of law (though it may be of help), in most instances it reassures the patient that the surgeon is not embarking on the procedure lightly. The informed consent thereby becomes a vehicle which helps prepare the patient psychologically by cementing his understanding, involvement, and trust.

CONCLUSION

I have outlined what I consider to be important goals in the psychological preparation of the patient for major surgery and have described how I attempt to achieve these goals. I believe the surgeon accepts an awesome responsibility when he undertakes major surgery and should never forget "primum non nocere" (firstly, do no harm). If the patient is allowed to perceive this attitude in his surgeon, trust and confidence will follow.

NAME:

UNIT #:

ADDENDUM TO
PRESBYTERIAN HOSPITAL INFORMED CONSENT
BY ALFRED JARETZKI III, M.D.

1. Dr. Jaretzki has explained to me, and to my satisfaction, the operation he and his assistants are going to perform and he has outlined the reasons for his recommendations.
2. I clearly understand that I do not have to undergo this operation, that there are alternatives available to me, and that the alternatives have been explained to me including the option that I not have the operation at this time.
3. I understand that the words "No Restrictions" indicate that Dr. Jaretzki has my permission to make minor or major alterations in the operative plan, depending on the findings and circumstances, from discontinuation of the procedure to major resectional surgery.
4. I am aware that the practice of medicine and surgery is not an exact science and that therefore reputable practitioners cannot guarantee results. I acknowledge that no guarantee or assurance or warranty has been made by Dr. Jaretzki regarding the results of the operation which I have herein requested and authorized.
5. I understand that there are risks (including the risk of permanent disability and death) associated with this operation and Dr. Jaretzki has informed me, to the extent to which I want to be informed, in this regard.
6. I understand that there may be complications associated with this operation, both intraoperatively and postoperatively (including any major illness or injury involving the nervous system, heart, lungs, liver, kidneys, extremities, etc.), and Dr. Jaretzki has informed me in this regard to the extent that I wish to be informed as well.
7. And finally, Dr. Jaretzki has answered to my satisfaction all the questions I have asked him.

WITNESS _____   SIGNED: _____ (PATIENT)

DATED: _____

In my opinion the patient understands the significance of the informed consent which has been given.

_____

Alfred Jaretzki III, M.D.

Revised May 1985

Part II
DEHUMANIZATION AND LOSS OF CONTROL
IN THE INSTITUTIONAL ENVIRONMENT

4

THE HOSPITAL ENVIRONMENT

HENRY ARANOW

This discussion will be restricted to problems that may have to be faced by competent, adult patients. I start with the assumption that, when a competent adult patient agrees to enter the hospital for surgical treatments he expects that these will probably be of benefit to him.* My thoughts concern those features common to many hospitals which may weaken the patient's conviction that he has embarked on the correct course for himself by provoking antipathetic reactions. The mere exposition of many of these indicates their remedies.

The features described may occur singly, or several at a time, at varying times during the patient's course from his decision to accept an operation as the optimal treatment for his particular problem, to his receipt of his last financial statement from the hospital and/or his medical attendants. For convenience, these are listed under four general headings but they may interdigitate and have a synergistic reaction with others.

These general headings are:
(1) DEPERSONALIZATION
(2) FOREIGNNESS
(3) LOSS OF AUTONOMY (CONTROL)
(4) FEARSOME EXPERIENCES

---

*I find the attempt to use pronouns that relate to both sexes cumbersome. Throughout this paper, he, his, and him are to be considered as indicating either he or she, his or hers, or him or her.

27

DEPERSONALIZATION

Impersonality is an almost invariable feature of any large, organizational operation. The concerns of the ill patient, however, are such that he seeks and hopes for procedures designed to help him as an individual.

Fortunate, indeed, is the patient who knows his surgeon more than casually, and has a friendly relationship with the surgeon's secretary. For many patients, depersonalization begins as soon as the decision to operate is made. Present financial pressures on hospitals have led them to endeavor to make certain, when an admission is not an emergency, that there is some person or agency responsible for, and capable of, paying the expenses of the hospitalization. Guided through the forms by a friend, the patient often finds them less alienating. When administered and executed by a busy clerk in a hospital admitting office, the listing of social security number, names and addresses of relatives, insurance companies and the numbers of the relevant policies—the admissions process—often makes the patient experience emotions similar to those reported by military draftees on induction. When a prepayment is requested, the suspicion may arise in the patient's mind that the hospital is more interested in getting paid than in helping him. If the execution of the admitting financial and insurance documents results in a long waiting time in the admitting office, irritation is added to the feeling of depersonalization. Since most patients are anxious at the prospect of hospitalization and operation their mood, when they finally reach the floor on which they will be lodged, is often far from good.

All too often, as the patient and accompanying family or friends emerge from the elevator the ward clerk calls to the head nurse to say, either, "Dr. Doe's gall-bladder has just arrived" or "622 is here and ready for admission." On busy floors and services the staff may not announce the patient by his name or refer to him by it when talking about him to others, but will use designations like those noted above to convey his identity to the listener. When this habit is ingrained, many of the staff never take the trouble to learn the patient's name, or to address him by it.

The courtesy of checking the patient's name on the door of his room, or on the foot of his bed, and greeting him by it, is often neglected by house staff and, to a lesser degree, by nurses. Technicians are usually more careful, since they often wish to make certain that the procedure they are about to perform has, indeed, been ordered for the patient before them. People are surprisingly grateful when floor personnel greet them by name, or wish them "Good morning" or "Good evening" etc., even when there is no procedure immediately impending. This courtesy helps to restore their frequently damaged sense of individuality.

FOREIGNNESS

Those who have visited hospitals in Third World countries are not surprised to find that most of the natives, when admitted to hospital, find themselves in a truly foreign world. Those of us who spend our lives working in and around hospitals in our own country may not be fully aware of how foreign the hospital environment is to many of its inhabitants. This is true for people from many backgrounds and is not limited to those from one of the ethnic subgroups.

Most hospitals were designed by architects who were primarily concerned about making them efficient places in which physicians, nurses, and other health care personnel could work. Esthetic considerations and patient preferences rarely weighed in making these designs, and studies of patient preferences are only now being undertaken. The subspecialty of "Hospital Design" is a relatively new one. The patient's perception of the hospital environment as strange may play a role in the disorientation that may plague elderly, hospitalized patients, and has certainly been an important factor in the movement back toward home delivery and, more specifically, in the design of hospital-attached "birthing centers."

Added to the architectural strangeness is the arcane jargon spoken by many of those who work in hospitals, from transporters to service chiefs. "ERs, ORs, CCUs, IVs, CAT scans, ultrasonograms, EEGs, EKGs, EMGs" fill the air around patients, who are moving from one location to another, and the conversations of physicians and nurses who discuss the patient's problem in his presence. Busy staff members may neglect to explain these terms even to the patients who are scheduled to be the subjects for one or more of them. When discussions are directed to the patient, the medical staff often seem to have difficulty in keeping them in standard English.

LOSS OF CONTROL (AUTONOMY)

Since childhood, the majority of healthy patients have decided for themselves what they would eat, drink, and wear, and when they would arise from bed, and retire into it. Almost all of these decisions are taken out of the patient's hands when he enters a hospital. Even if he has missed his preceding meal, and is thirsty, he will generally not be allowed either to eat or drink until his doctor leaves an order for it. His sleeping hours must fit the hospital routines, and it is usually hospital rules that determine when his bedside light must be turned out.

Shortly after admission to the hospital, a patient is usually relieved of his regular garments which are taken from him—often stored in some unknown and distant place—and he is asked to don clothing designed to make it easy for attendants to put on and take off, and to perform the necessary tests. Esthetics seem to have received no consideration in their styling, and many of them cause embarrassment in patients whose sole body covering they constitute.

In many parts of the hospital, after he has been instructed in the manipulation of the several bells and buttons near his bed, a metallic P.A. transmitted voice speaks to a patient, rather than a voice emerging from a visible fellow human being.

Once settled in his bed, he may be abruptly snatched from it. In many instances, even though he may have walked into the hospital under his own power, he is told to sit in a wheelchair, or lie on a stretcher, which is then taken by a transporter to a destination which, all too often, has not been fully discussed with him before he's on the move toward it.

Physicians, medical students, and technicians may draw blood from him with no more than a pro forma request for permission, and even this is often forgotten.

Should the patient demur at any of these happenings, or demand an answer to his reasonable questions before being subjected to them, he runs the risk of being considered "uncooperative," with all the merely guessed at consequences that he fears may follow.

Most of the hospital's staff have not, themselves, been subjected to many of the tests that they order/perform on patients. In tests involving ionizing radiation, the patient is usually alone in the room, observed either through a radioopaque window, or on a TV screen, by the persons performing the test. One does not have to suffer from claustrophobia to experience anxiety when one's head is held immobile, surrounded by a whirring machine of large size, during a CAT scan. During a lung scan the registering device is placed very close to the patient's chest, and he is told to refrain from moving. Since such patients not infrequently already have respiratory symptoms, the psychological impact of the test tends to exacerbate them. The cyclotron is so huge that its weight would obviously easily crunch an elephant. A patient lying alone, under it, during his therapy, cannot help but wonder what would happen if some of the controls that lift and lower it went awry. When these tests are explained to the patient while his consent is being gained, the staff person is usually focusing on the fact that the radiation dosage involved is nondamaging and that the procedure involves no pain. The frightening strangeness of the patient's finding himself inside one of these pieces of apparatus is often not appreciated nor referred to, nor is the sense of helplessness he may then feel addressed.

Finally, the ultimate loss of control is being subjected to general anesthesia during which even one's breathing may no longer be under one's own control. Many patients have been made anxious by stories of what they may reveal as they go under or emerge from anesthesia.

After surgery, the medication prescribed to relieve pain may be ordered at intervals that the patient may feel are inappropriately long. As those familiar with the pharmacology of analgesics know, there is a great deal of arbitrariness in the choice or size of dose and the intervals at which it is to be administered. Much of the time when a house officer prescribes an analgesic over the telephone, he may be unaware of the patient's pain threshold, his degree of anxiety, and often, his body size. All who have worked in hospitals, however, know with what scepticism patients' statements of the inadequacy of analgesia are often received. Here again, to suffer pain the relief of which is quite removed from the patient's control, adds to his feeling of loss of autonomy.

His postoperative activity, too, is determined by others and he often feels that their explanations either of the imperatives to increase it at a given time, or to restrain it when he feels them easily within his capacity, are often so brief as to be inadequate.

FEARSOME EXPERIENCES

Under this heading I shall list only a few examples. I shall not include events that are a necessary part of the patient's therapy but only remediable and avoidable problems. Some do not directly involve the patient but may involve those visiting him. However, each is relevant to the general perception of the hospital environment held by much of the public.

An unduly large number of these events occur in elevators. In spite of constant efforts on the part of administration and staff, many people working in the hospital do not discontinue private conversations with colleagues about particular patients when they enter elevators in which patients' visitors may be riding. Some of the episodes I have personally witnessed have not only dealt with unfortunate mishaps that had occurred in the hospital but also have identified the particular patient involved. They are often dramatic enough to interest other hospital staff workers, and of a character to arouse alarm even in the passing visitor, and much more in the relatives of the patient. In some elevators there are both patients and hospital workers, and even their evident presence does not deter some from discussing matters that may distress their auditors.

The evident psychological impact of bedside ward rounds has long been known. (I was myself a member of a group to which the ward attending, at the patient's bedside at a time when the patient was in the early stages of his illness, said, "I have never seen a patient with this disease recover.") Group discussions about other patients in the room may be misunderstood by the patient as being about his problem. It is encouraging that, in recent years, the bedside examination of the patient has been increasingly restricted to verifying important details about his history, his reports of his current symptoms, and his physical examination, while deferring discussions of diagnosis, indicated laboratory examinations, and therapy to meetings in adjoining areas. I hasten to add, however, that the inclusion of the patient on wards rounds also has a positive effect on his morale if the discussions are properly restricted; he often interprets them as indications of interest in his problems.

There are many routines, not necessarily part of the environment, that are so frequently associated with it in patient's minds that they merit mention.

The lowly bedpan is one. Bowel evacuation on a hospital bedpan is, for many patients, a difficult balancing act. Not a few untoward cardiovascular reactions have followed straining at stool. What has not been adequately appreciated is that less energy is required to move one's bowels on a bedside commode than on a bedpan.

The stress imposed by the order "strict bed rest" is often not realized. When I was a house officer, this was the routine order for all patients who were admitted with a recent myocardial infarction. No one who has not experienced it realizes how stressful it is to have one's teeth cleaned by a person who has had no dental hygienic training, but "strict bed rest" did not allow the patient to brush his own teeth, and it was done by the nurse assigned to that patient; other restrictions on even minimal activity may be even more onerous. As you know, "strict bed rest" has since been found to be indicated for only a very small minority of patients with myocardial infarctions.

Sensory deprivation can produce serious psychological disturbances. A particularly striking example of the untoward side effects of immobilization and sensory deprivation was seen by me in a number of patients in the Eye hospital. Until relatively recent research showed how meaningless it was, patients recovering from operative repairs of retinal detachments had their eyes patched, and were told that it was very important for them to keep their eyes immobile. This stress added to that caused by their concern about their vision and produced more than a few acute upper gastrointestinal hemorrhages. We now know that during rapid eye movement sleep eye movements more violent than voluntary ones are usual; but the old routine was still in effect in the postoperative orders of some surgeons.

Special problems are evident in a number of "Special Hospital Areas." Many of them are combinations of problems already referred to: in the *Tank Respirator* sensory deprivation is a major threat, and similar considerations apply to *Isolation Units*. Specifically related to the Open Heart Recovery Room are: an open room in which the patient can witness the problems of other patients unless his curtains are drawn; in many instances curtains are kept pulled back to permit better observation of several patients by a limited number of nurses; immobility, enforced by cables, wires, and catheters; the background humming of oxygen equipment, the flashing lights of the cardiac monitors, and sleep deprivation. Many similar conditions are found in Coronary Care Units, to which the ringing of an alarm bell is often added. A cardiac arrest, and the subsequent attempts at resuscitation by the large group such an event usually mobilizes, is often in full view of other patients in the unit. Since the patient is aware of the fact that he is probably at risk for a similar occurrence, such viewings are often very disturbing.

In the *Operating Room* some patients under general anesthesia have recalled conversations held about them by surgeons and anesthetists at times when they were presumed to be completely unconscious. This finding should be kept in mind by those who work in them.

The *Surgical Recovery Room* for patients who are emerging from general anesthesia after major operations is often filled with patients in several states of alertness. Some may have fully emerged from the effects of their anesthetic and are being held in the Recovery Room until their floors are ready to receive them. Scenes take place before their eyes that may make more literate patients think they are witnessing scenes in Dante's *Inferno.* Staff members often communicate with one another by calling aloud across the room in a language only parts of which may be intelligible to the conscious patient. Personal experience in these gives me the conviction that psychic trauma to the patient in these units is frequent: patients' diagnoses and pathological findings are often discussed as though there were no auditors other than physicians and nurses.

As indicated above, a mere listing and exposition of many of these problems leads to an immediate appreciation of their remedies. Most of them require no more than awareness by the personnel who are in contact with patients, and a reasonable concern for the untoward effects of conduct which is under voluntary control. Some corrections will require easily effected changes in routine, others will demand more forethought on the part of hospital architects, and understanding by those who must approve their plans.

5

COMMON COMPLAINTS ABOUT INTENSIVE CARE—BY PATIENTS OR FAMILY MEMBERS

HENRIK H. BENDIXEN

Modern intensive care has a brief history, having its origin in the years around 1960. It was stimulated by the successes in providing artificial ventilation for polio victims during the epidemics of the 1950s, and to a greater extent by the growing needs of intrathoracic surgery. Intensive care was required for the successful practice of open-heart surgery and other major surgery.

Although the results of intensive care were highly encouraging in its first decade, the intensive care units were high intensity users of both technology and manpower, resulting in high costs. Soon, other complaints were added, most of them addressing the dehumanizing features of intensive care, the wasteful heroic efforts undertaken by the physician in charge, and the lack of dignity imposed on the dying. To the complaint that intensive care is often dehumanizing, one must agree; it is difficult to avoid causing patients to feel that this happens in view of the necessary interventions in modern intensive care. For a patient, it is dehumanizing to have an endotracheal tube in place, being attached to a mechanical respirator, having tubes in stomach and bladder, as well as lines of various types in veins and arteries, both for monitoring and infusions. Add to the setting the presence of blinking lights, beeping alarms, and a bedside crowded with electronics, with the patient literally pinned down in bed, disenfranchised, more or less deprived of the ability to participate and communicate; and often being talked about instead of being talked to. Again, dehumanizing effects are exceedingly difficult to avoid, when care becomes intensive in our modern units. At the same time, this is no excuse for not fully understanding the patient's predicament and making earnest efforts to treat the patient with every consideration and to minimize these negative effects.

Does the patient suffer under these circumstances? Sometimes unquestionably yes! However, in a well-run intensive care unit suffering should be the exception rather than the rule, because one of the fringe benefits of having patients on a mechanical respirator, with controlled oxygenation, is that they can be kept free of pain, well sedated, and partially obtunded to a degree which can be titrated to individual requirements. Under the circumstances of intensive care, even long-term use of narcotic drugs seems to cause no addiction, and the patients can be weaned from any drug dependence once the underlying trauma or illness is brought under control.

Few if any patients need to suffer in the modern intensive care unit, if available drugs are used intelligently. The drawbacks or side-effects are few, and the major inconvenience may be the patient's decreased ability to communicate. Almost invariably, family members appreciate the situation fully and agree that less communication is a small price to pay for knowing that at least the patient is comfortable.

Another frequent complaint about intensive care units is that futile heroic efforts are often undertaken by the physicians working there. Looked at superficially, this accusation may seem correct. However, a more careful analysis of the situation will reveal greater complexity than first meets the eye.

The problem is that often patients with end-stage diseases of various kinds are admitted to the intensive care unit, intubated and put on mechanical respirators. Only in retrospect is it discovered that the underlying disease is end-stage and that the moment of death is approaching. How does one recognize patients with end-stage disease? Importantly, such patients cannot be spotted at the door to the intensive care unit, nor can they be identified with any certainty, in the emergency room when they arrive in distress, with pending cardiorespiratory failure. Such patients must be given the benefit of all doubts, and if that means intubation and mechanical ventilation in the intensive care unit, so be it. End-stage disease can only be recognized reliably at the level of primary care by the family physician, who must then undertake to plan for the patient's remaining life span in consultation with the patient and the family.

Parenthetically, a social trend of major importance is the change in the location of dying. Up until 1950, the majority of deaths took place in the home of the dying individual. By contrast, now in the 1980s, at least 80 percent of the population are dying in institutions, mostly in acute hospitals. It is enormously costly and quite inappropriate, as well as undesirable from the patient's point of view, for most deaths to take place in the acute hospital, certainly in its intensive care units.

A related complaint is that treatment should be stopped more often than is currently the case, especially when one recognizes that the mortality for a certain disease is very high. There are several answers to this complaint. First, statistics are of little use when dealing with the care of the individual patient, because uncertainty remains over whether the patient is going to be among the relatively few survivors or whether efforts will have been in vain. For the longest time if the disease is potentially reversible, it is certainly not possible to deny the patient the chance, even though it may be one in ten or less. Second, room must always be allowed for the possibility that the assessment of the patient may be incorrect, and that the patient to everyone's surprise may leave the intensive care unit alive and well. This is not a common event, but it happens. Third, with an incapacitated patient, the patient's family and their spokesperson, if one can be identified, must be informed and consulted about the management that seems in the patient's best interest. And this may take a little time. A striking point is this: it is almost never important to arrive at a disposition within minutes or hours. Time is almost never of the essence and, surprisingly often, the natural time course of the illness will eventually reveal itself, often making it unnecessary for physicians and the family to go through agonizing decision making. One should always consider the advisability of resuscitating the patient in case of cardiorespiratory arrest, certainly when the patient is elderly or very ill. The decision should be put in writing in the patient's record.

In this context, it should be noted how important it is to keep the relationship with the family the best possible. They should be kept well-informed. They should be told the truth, but without being overloaded with information and without having bad news sprung on them more suddenly than is necessary. One should also recognize that in a final illness there will often be a display of guilt among family members, accounting for some of the difference in approaches to what should be done for the patient. Often those who are most insistent that everything be done for the patient in the face of a hopeless situation, feel guilty about having previously ignored the dying patient.

In its roughly twenty-year history, modern intensive care units have proven to be cost-effective, but not always so. Our greatest current problem is the overuse of the intensive care unit in the care of end-stage disease. But to repeat the previously reached conclusion, it takes effective primary care to protect the intensive care unit against an inappropriate admission of a patient in end-stage disease, a patient who should spend the final hours and days under less dehumanizing and more dignified circumstances than the modern ICU has to offer.

6

ETHICAL CONSIDERATIONS IN INTENSIVE CARE

Allen I. Hyman

When I was in school, whenever we discussed the questions of medical ethics we referred to those that pertained to social behavior and to honest conduct and to the expected courtesies of physicians toward one another. Today, these issues seem superficial, simple, even frivolous compared to the ethical quandaries facing us. We question whether we are now at a historical turning point in the development of human and ethical values. We know that the rapid advances in science have suddenly given physicians new and increasing power that enables us to dramatically affect the lives of patients. At the same time, we see the material expenditure for this new power to be of such a magnitude that it can create imbalances in our economy. We ask: Must we change or even stretch the ethical principles we have held so long, so that these scientific achievements do not distort the economic framework of our society. Triage focuses directly on this key question.

The term triage stems from the French word "trier." Originally, it meant to select or to choose different grades of commodities, such as coffees or berries. In our time, triage has acquired a medical quality and refers to a screening process of patients to determine their order of priority for treatment. Usually, the term is used in the context of describing the management of a disaster, the division of casualties into three groups. In the first group are those who would not likely survive even with treatment; in the second group are those who would probably recover even without treatment; in the priority group are those who must be treated in order to survive. Triage has now taken on a new dimension. It is used to describe medical decisions that must be made when the demand for medical resources, material, space, and manpower exceeds their supply. Medical triage ultimately implies the process of choosing one person over another.

Nowhere in a modern hospital are our moral and ethical values tested more than in intensive care units. In the ICU's the issues of life and death are placed in sharper focus than elsewhere, mainly because here are the resources to keep people, who would otherwise be dead, alive almost indefinitely. While there have been extraordinary changes in the last two decades in the way we care for critically ill patients, this progress has not come about through any major breakthrough in our basic understanding of disease processes, nor have there been fundamental differences applied in their treatment. Rather, these changes have come about through the orderly application one-by-one of advances in technology and in personnel management. Space age science has literally been brought to the bedside and gradually applied to patients within this special environment. In the ICU, there is a concentration of skilled, proficient, and specially trained people plus an extensive array of complex costly equipment.

But our ability to sustain life or, as it may seem at times, prolong death in the intensive care unit has created enormous dilemmas—social, economic, and ethical. Many complex issues are raised in the intensive care unit: The right to life, definition of death, and dying with dignity. In relation to triage, this chapter considers another enigma: Who shall live when not all can live? There is a risk that framing health care issues in ethical expressions can lead us to inaction. We might elevate the discussion and debate of these thorny problems to so high a level that inevitably there is no solution. The "Bottom Line, Hard Nosed" medical economists often admonish the romantic idealists of the 1960s for ignoring the practical realities of scarcities. A generation ago, when less than 5 percent of our annual economic output was spent for health, medical care was declared by our national political leaders to be a right and those who might benefit were promised all they would need. Now we spend more than 10 percent of what we produce on medical care and we have grown cautious and restrained about our expectations of allocating any more of our income to health. Today the bottom line health question is not simply is it necessary, but more to the point, can we afford it? Cost effectiveness has become part of political rhetoric. To consider cost effectiveness in terms of health has created an ethical dilemma for all of us.

For the first time in our nation's history, we are debating the issues of planned allocation of health care, or to put it bluntly, we are discussing the rationing of medicine. The accelerated cost of health care, whether justified or not, is beginning to crowd out other essential functions and services of a normal society. All levels of government must carefully rank their needs for health services against those for defense, safety, schools, parks and libraries, and so forth. Some say we have reached this precipice because for too long we have been guided by the moral principle expressed medically as doing everything possible for everyone in need regardless of who pays. Free health care, free in the sense of meaning not directly paid for by the person who receives the care, has become a basic political right. And since what we perceive to be free, we consume avidly, sometimes lavishly and even wastefully, we should not be surprised that health care costs are rising more rapidly than most other elements of our economy. In Great Britain, it has been speculated that since the ultimate need for free health care for each person is infinite, this demand is everlasting and can never be met. The longer you live, the more you need; the more you get the longer you live and so on and so on. However much we spend, the demand will inevitably rise to exceed it. It necessarily follows that if our finite resources can never equal the demand for free medical care, painful decisions will and must be made at some level of government or institutions affecting individuals that ultimately will lead to the ethical dilemma of who shall live when not all can live and who shall decide. In some western countries, this quandary is answered by the queue. As a government policy, the number of specialists, hospitals, and equipment has been deliberately kept so low that while no one is explicitly denied care, for many access to the system takes so long or is so complicated that the process serves as de facto rationing. People may die before they are admitted into the system. And as one cynic put it, in the health care system, death is the ultimate economy.

This country may never bring its medical care expenditures under control unless it is willing to accept the notion that some medical benefits are not worth the cost even when health is at stake. Locally, within the hospital we can see competition for scarce resources. The ICU embodies and, in fact, provides for doctors the means to serve their basic inclination to do everything feasible for their patients. But rising ICU costs must inevitably put pressure on expenditures for other worthwhile but seemingly less crucial or dramatic hospital programs. To be sure, to prevent the distortion of health care goals within the hospital, intensive care facilities should be used only for those patients for whom there is a reasonable expectation of their receiving benefits from these expensive resources. Too often, in many hospitals, patients with terminal disease, or with irreversible brain damage, spend their last days tethered to life support systems in an ICU.

Deeply ingrained within each of us is the moral principle that each human being has infinite and equal value, that we as physicians must preserve and dignify human life, that life is indivisible, that a single day is no less precious than a decade. So how should we act? Must we bend our moral convictions if we accept the nature and implications of limited and scarce resources? As physicians, we know we must give whatever is necessary to those in need. But we now understand that giving all to some may lead to having less for the others. The cost for one baby's ICU care for three months could feed more than a thousand hungry children. How then should we act?

Our best hope, for the time being, is to have each individual with responsibility for others make the best case for his own constituency. In the context of the ICU, the patient's own personal physician should act as the patient's advocate. With the patient and his family, the physician need consider only what is best for his patient. He presents his claim to the director of the ICU. The medical director of the ICU is responsible for carrying out the policies of the unit. He should serve his constituency, namely all patients who require the support services of the ICU. The director's decision on the distribution of scarce resources should be impartial to any consideration other than the patient's need for and likely benefit from intensive care. The director is responsible for planning, so that the ICU's resources may become less expensive, less scarce, and it follows there would be fewer occasions when patients would have to compete for the ICU beds. The director presents his case to the hospital administrator, who in turn decides on the priorities within the hospital. Who gets the last empty bed in the ICU? Should it be the saint or the scoundrel? Should we in fact consider, as some have suggested, distributing medical resources according to a measure or assessment of the patient's merit, worthiness, or value to society? Or should it be left to chance to an impartial process available to those with equivalent need?

I believe that when claims are identical and incompatible, a system of random selection is most likely to promote the highest human values. Each person has then been given an equal chance to receive that which all cannot have. Occasionally the scoundrel may gain the last ICU bed, and the saint loses. But this system is better than one in which the scoundrel becomes the moral assessor and inevitably decides who shall live and who shall not.

Under our political system, ultimately we are responsible to determine the proportion of our economic output we wish to devote to medical needs, even to particular medical programs. We must recognize and courageously face these new challenges. We must come down from the lofty peaks and ivory towers where ethicists discuss amongst themselves abstract principles and theories. We must confront and attack these hard issues with the same zeal, practicality, and intellect that brought us our scientific achievements.

7

INTENSIVE CARE: THE PATIENT

RUSSELL LYNES

L ast May my gall bladder exploded, to use my layman's vernacular, in what I gather was a particularly nasty way.* A few days after I had been returned from intensive care to my room in Harkness, Dr. Herter, who had operated on me, asked if I would be willing to "give a paper" about my experience as a patient in an intensive care unit. By then I had gathered some, but apparently not all or I wouldn't be here, of what pass for my wits, and I said I would be glad to if he thought my doing so would be useful—an opportunity in a sense for me to return my kind of professional services for his life-sustaining kind. He left with me a photocopy of a hand-written outline of a symposium, an early draft, and asked, if I had any comments or suggestions, to let him know.

I read the outline with an interest I might not have had if I had not been on a knife edge of which I was just then becoming aware. On the printed program, I was listed under the subhead of "Intensive Care" as "the patient," and identified as "writer, patient, New York." On the first draft of this program my role was more descriptive. I was, more particularly, to be the patient in a session on "loss of identity and control in intensive care." My initial reaction to seeing this in the outline was, "Well, I'll be damned." Loss of identity and control was news to me.

Not quite. I had flashes of recollection of being in what I was later told was intensive care (I didn't know where I had been), but they were no

---

*According to Dr. Hamilton Southworth: "Acute cholecystitis without stones leading to gangrene of gall bladder and bacteremia, cholototomy, post-op pneumonitis, post-op confusion."

more than flashes—split seconds, like heat lightning at night, and sounds that were like the snap of gun fire and distant voices and a few whispers. I could not describe the room; I cannot describe it now, though my sense of it is of a pervasive whiteness, which may be merely the contrast from the darkness my mind wandered in or the kind of whiteness the sky assumes when it is seen from a deep cleft in the earth. During some of these flashes I was aware (or I think I was, though what was fantasy then and persists as such and what was fact I have no way even now to distinguish)—I was aware of a row of gowned figures of indeterminate sex across the room from me, a long way off. I think of them as white, but then everything was white and melted together, a froth of sheets and gowns and a row of furry snowmen in an antiseptic snow fort. If this seems to you too literary a visual metaphor and hyperbole besides, let me remind you that, as you can see, I wear glasses, I am both myopic and astigmatic and when I am deprived of my glasses, as I obviously was in intensive care, even a giant refrigerator melts into fuzziness at ten feet.

Indeed my experience in intensive care was hyperbole, an exaggeration, dreamlike in its disunity, its suggestiveness, its parody of reality, its contrasts of disembodiment (floating) on the one hand, and exaggerated physicality on the other, its aloofness from pain and its intensity of reaction to touch.

Let me be as specific as I can, allowing not only for the distorting haze of the occasion itself but the blurrings of the passage of time. I have let writing this paper go. I had no stomach for sorting out my feelings and observations while I was recovering my physical strength, and though I was aware of no wounds of mind or spirit from the experience then (or now), I was more interested in when I would be rid of the bile bag attached to my abdomen and when the strength would be back in my legs than I was in reliving my misadventure on a typewriter. I was also delighted by the excuse not to write (knowing it would be temporary) and to spend my time reading novels by writers I admire . . . and some I found I didn't. My close shave did not lead me to speculations on death but to literary explorations of life, some grim some otherwise.

I can be specific about only a very few things that I did or felt or imagined happened to me in intensive care in a state, I learned when I read Dr. Kornfeld's diagnosis on a medicare form some weeks later, was "delirium."

There are just four specific moments that I recall. I ripped out the catheter that had at some time of which I have no recollection been inserted. I did so because I felt I was being tied down by my penis for reasons I did not understand and certainly did not like. I recall a voice whispering by my ear, "Let's try it here," and then a needle (or was it a tube?) was inserted near my right shoulder. My reaction was, "What do they mean *try?* Don't they know what they're doing?" I was, I thought, being experimented on. I remember taking a swipe with my fist at—was it a nurse or was it a physician? I don't recall, but the object of my fury or, more likely, my fright, was a female. I don't know if I hit her, but she jumped and let out a small cry. (The only other time I can remember swinging at anyone was in my early childhood when I hit a bigger boy than me with a toy snow shovel because he rubbed my face with snow and put snow down my neck. I knocked his wind out and when he stopped gasping he cried. His crying scared the daylights out of me.) I remember a man's voice saying from what seemed a great distance, "Do you know who you are?" and "Do you know where you are?" This seemed to me silly and rather insulting. How should I not know who I was? I remember answering but not what I said. I did not know I was in an intensive care unit; I did know I was in a hospital. I may have said "New York Hospital," where years before I had come to on the operating table and was reassured that "it was all over." I had had an operation on my upper spine. I was surprised but not frightened.

There was one other moment that I recall and which I expect I'll never forget. It cannot have lasted more than a few seconds, and I cannot accurately describe it. There was a moment, a very quiet moment, when I was deep in the dark crevass by myself when the thought crossed my mind gently and without alarm that it would be very easy to die—as easy as not to die. But I had the choice. I was not in the least frightened. It seemed a very simple matter, as simple and effortless as closing my eyes or opening a door. I do not remember making a decision. Apparently I did. If not my mind then my body made it for me.

I am sure that many of you could tell me why I remember nothing from the time I was put on a stretcher on leaving the emergency room until the confused incidents I have recounted from the intensive care unit and nothing from then until I came to my senses several days later in Harkness 758 with my wife standing by my bed. I have no recollection of the day before the operation when, I'm told, I was in room 758, nor of the anaesthetic nor of the recovery room. Whether these blank stretches (for they are completely blank) are from what I believe psychologists call "oblivescence of the disagreeable" or were induced by the drugs I was given or by my illness, I have no idea.

I also have no lessons or conclusions to draw from my experience that I can believe may be useful to you, though there are some insights into the nature of mortality that cannot but be useful to me. One does not get that close to death and know it (unlike the closeness to death we live with daily) without discovering that life is far more than just being alive, a cliché, a truism, and without suspecting that death may be as interesting as life, a suspicion I am happy to have left temporarily unresolved.

My experience as "writer, patient, New York" in intensive care might have been quite different, or anyway my attitude toward it, if I had been told that I would be operated on, that I was in serious trouble, that I would find myself coming to in a recovery room (I'd been in one a few times before and, like everyone else I know, hated it) if I had been warned that . . . and so on. The fact, I suppose, is that I was warned, was told, was reassured because I was for the most part in the humane and concerned hands of physicians and surgeons I trusted and who were my friends, one of them a friend of fifty years. There was no moment (admittedly there was a blizzard of confused moments) when I was worried about dying or about being in hands that were less than deeply concerned for my life. With a single exception, a doctor who seemed more interested in me as a potential future customer than as a present patient, I emerged from my experience in this hospital with a consummate respect for everyone who took care of me. I am sometimes short-tempered (as the woman I swung at in intensive care can testify; I apologize to her profoundly), but I am not vindictive, and if I were I'd have no grudge, no suspicion, no complaint to justify it. Someone made off from my room with a beautiful gold key chain that my wife had given me many years ago. My fault. I should have handed it over to "security," but my wits were elsewhere. It was the only thing I lost from my experience except for my gall bladder, eighteen useless pounds, my temper, my sanity (briefly), and my innocence.

8

CARDIAC SURGERY: FACING DEHUMANIZATION, LOSS OF CONTROL, AND ENVIRONMENTAL SHOCK

Henry M. Spotnitz

INTRODUCTION

Dehumanization is described in *Webster's Dictionary* as divesting of human qualities or personality. I believe that the degree to which we succeed in "dehumanizing" a patient is a measure of our failure as physicians. I am referring in this not to the physical animation of the individual, but to the inner perceptions of the health care team, particularly the physicians. For example, externally the patient who undergoes deep hypothermia and total circulatory arrest for complex cardiac surgery appears nearly dead. There is no heart beat, no external evidence of brain function; and brain wave activity is decreased. Much of the patient's blood may have been temporarily drained, and body temperature is lower than room temperature. But surely this patient is not dead, and any tendency to perceive this as death impairs our motivation to return the patient to health. Regardless of external appearance, in the operating room or intensive care unit, the cardiac surgeon strives to preserve the patient's life, health, welfare, and personal interests just as if the patient were alert. Therefore, I reject the concept of "dehumanization" and will not explicitly discuss it further.

Intensive care is a complex art which is optimized not only by effective delivery of medical care but also by attention to those details that impact on emotional well-being. Failure in this latter area results in a postoperative emotional aberration which in the extreme can disrupt other aspects of care and cause a life-threatening crisis. Recent evolution of postoperative care, however, appears to have made such problems less common after cardiac surgery. This reflects both better surgery and better understanding of the problem. Most patients now leave the Intensive Care Unit (ICU) within 72 hours after surgery. Air and particulate embolism and low output states are less common. Thus, frank neurologic dysfunction is also less common, and secondary triggering of bizarre emotional reactions has been reduced. Doctors and nurses have learned to decrease anxiety through skillful and systematic education of patients and families, sensitivity to patient concerns, and adequate communication. The importance of orientation to time, outside views, music, and television has been appreciated. Patients in the ICU are even occasionally allowed to sleep, but probably not enough.

BEFORE SURGERY

Before cardiac surgery, patients fear death, pain, permanent injury, loss of sanity, and loss of control. Depending on personal circumstances, economic factors and family welfare are also important issues. The level of conversation between surgeon and patient is importantly altered when the patient agrees to surgery. The need for surgery may come as a shock to previously healthy people who in short order are stricken with chest pain, admitted to hospital, and told after cardiac catheterization that they have surgical heart disease. Others undergo catheterization without really believing they are seriously ill, only to find that their disease is too critical to allow them to leave the hospital without surgery. This can be a difficult situation or a straightforward one. If the patient understands that his life is in jeopardy but that chances of surgical cure are excellent, surgery is usually chosen, sometimes hesitantly. If the patient refuses, deeper issues may be involved. Family arguments, loss of income during surgery and recovery, and deeper emotional issues may be relevant. The surgeon's role in this setting is to educate the patient and his immediate family and to work with other physicians trusted by the patient to provide gentle encouragement. Patients who are reluctant to agree to surgery should be given a reasonable time to reconsider and allowed to refuse if they are adult and competent. Patients who agree to surgery under excessive family or physician pressure are eternally ungrateful if results are less than perfect. I believe such patients manifest severe emotional conflict postoperatively more commonly than most. On the other hand, fear and anxiety before cardiac surgery are common and normal. A patient who is quoted an unusually high surgical mortality and accepts cheerfully may also be telling us something and needs to be carefully watched.

An important emotional problem for the surgeon is the patient who persistently refuses surgery out of fear but survives to become a high risk surgical emergency. If the patient died, or refused surgery to the grave, we would not personally have a problem. But patients often change their minds when death is imminent, and we are left to make the best of a difficult situation. I have cared for such a patient, a psychologist in his early fifties with unstable angina. He had flunked the Pritikin program and was on his way for chelation therapy by a local charlatan when he was suddenly stricken with severe symptoms. He came to the Emergency Room asking for me and died. Autopsy revealed a normal heart except for single vessel coronary disease. It would appear that he wanted surgical help when all other options ran out. Experiences like this present us with a serious moral dilemma that has no simple answers. We want to convince patients of the folly of excessive delay, but the patient's wishes and limitations still must be respected.

When a patient agrees to cardiac surgery, the physician must obtain what is somewhat ambiguously referred to as "Informed Consent." Our approach is to provide patients with educational materials, training programs, and extensive discussions of procedures, risks, and complications. Therapists, nurses, house staff, anesthesiologists, internists and my physician's assistant participate in patient education. But what do I do when my patient doesn't want to read the books and doesn't want to hear my patented preop lecture? Recently, a woman in her fifties was suddenly confronted with the need for valve replacement. She had critical aortic stenosis which was far out of proportion to the physical findings. She timorously agreed to urgent surgery, proposed by her internist. I went to see her, and she was obviously frightened. Her only living relatives are siblings, living in Florida. I told her I agreed that her aortic valve needed to be replaced. In order to do this, we would use a heart-lung machine. "That's too technical," she said, and would allow me to offer no further information. "But wait!" I thought, "I haven't told you about the risks! I haven't told you about bleeding, heart block, embolism, heart attack, stroke!" "Would you like to know about the different kinds of valves and their problems?" I asked. "No," she said. She signed surgical consent with no further verbal exchange and subsequently has presented no problems, surgically or emotionally. Was this patient's

Consent Informed? Were she and I within our rights and responsibilities? What would have happened if she had suffered a disabling stroke? In this area, as in others, we still have much to learn.

How should we talk to patients about surgical mortality? In this context, is "10 percent probability of death" the same as "90 percent chance of survival?" Does "90 percent chance of survival" mean the same thing if most patients have a 99 percent chance of survival? If most patients have a predicted 1 percent mortality and Patient A has a predicted 10 percent mortality, should this be expressed as 10 percent mortality, 9 percent greater than most patients, or ten times greater than most patients? Is the use of percentages too abstract for some patients? Is it perhaps more meaningful in some instances to say "this is a good (or bad) situation and if we don't encounter unexpected problems, things should go well?"

Obviously, patients are individuals. In conversing with them, we are not just exchanging verbal information, but also emotional information. Patients want to know if their surgeon is competent and trustworthy and if he will go to The Wall for them if there is trouble. They want to know if the surgeon understands and respects them as well. They usually want to be kept well informed or have someone in their family kept informed about their state of health. Much of this is communicated by how we state things and how responsive we are as much as by what we say. The details of procedures and forms are much less significant in a climate of trust, and the patient's emotional well-being is promoted by confidence in the health care team. These are the goals. Success in achieving them has as much to do with sensitivity and personal style as all forms of human relations.

INTENSIVE CARE

In the ICU, the patient's preoperative level of anxiety is carried forward and altered by the course of events. The patient is bombarded by new sensations, altered body image, loss of sleep, and altered personal relationships. New sensations include pain, asphyxiation, and paroxysmal coughing during endotracheal suctioning. Patients are newly equipped with nasogastric, urinary drainage, and chest tubes. Residual paralysis and anesthesia are also problems as intraoperative drugs are metabolized. The patient's body image is altered. He cannot talk or breathe for himself, he cannot eat, he cannot void, except passively, and he receives nutrition and fluids insensibly. A pacemaker may be necessary to maintain a beating heart. Occasionally, blood pumps and dialysis are needed to maintain life. In addition, coughing and motion may be accompanied by pain from unanticipated sources.

Other anxiety-provoking experiences occur as well. These include misinterpreted sounds from malfunctioning monitors and misinterpreted casual remarks about other patients. The list also includes correctly interpreted and unfortunate remarks at the bedside as well as correct observation of nearby critically ill patients. An occasional, and unfortunately unavoidable, bonus is the chance to witness a full blown cardiac arrest and resuscitation. Families are frequently upset by the appearance of their loved one in the ICU, so that even the support of traditional family interactions may be disrupted. Patients at this stage desperately need emotional support and the comfort of human interaction. The more severely ill they are and the longer they are ill, the more they need this support. At times, this may be extremely difficult for the health care team, particularly if the patient's prognosis is bad, or if we feel personal responsibility for a bad surgical result. But emotional support and communication are essential at this stage if the chances for recovery are to be optimized.

For most patients, the passage of time after ICU admission brings rapid restoration of mental and physical health. For some, reduction of the fear of death seems to remove a lock on the anxiety and emotional turmoil festering before surgery. For others, initial elation at survival of surgery gives way to depression over the realization that a life-threatening illness has been experienced and that external help was needed for survival. Many poignant and bizarre behavior patterns may be seen in the two weeks after cardiac surgery. Mild-mannered patients may become physically abusive; brave, strong individuals may become weak and frightened. Some patients may decide to leave the hospital, as did one of our aortic valve recipients who walked out on the third postoperative day, trailing his telemeter behind him.

For most cardiac surgical patients, emotional reactions to surgery are moderate and easily managed by discussion and reassurance. For others, pharmacologic management and psychiatric consultation may be necessary. Through it all, communication is essential. The patient is entitled to understand the course of the illness and the measures being taken to control it. The patient is entitled to express satisfaction or dissatisfaction, whether appropriate or inappropriate. At the same time, we must avoid the tendency to force unwanted or emotionally damaging information on the patient or family.

In the last analysis, things go better when we can remember the human and personal qualities of our patients in the face of the complex events and dramatic changes that surround successful cardiac surgery.

Part III
IMPACT OF SURGERY
ON BODY IMAGE AND FUNCTION

9

DISFIGUREMENT: WHAT PRICE SURGICAL CARE OR PALLIATION?

John Conley

There are certain axioms that must be recognized in order to make a realistic assessment of the above proposition. The variables contained in the treatment of potentially fatal neoplasms in the area of the head and neck disrupt any guarantees for cure or local control or against systemic spread. A speculative hope is established within the framework of general biological neoplastic behavior and actuarial statistics on survival. One can be certain that extensive cancers in this area, if untreated or if unsuccessfully treated, will cause pain, disfigurement, loss of physiological function, and finally kill the patient. These progressive physical burdens unquestionably diminish both the quality of life and the meaning of life for the patient. It is in the midst of these stark axioms that a program of treatment must be developed.

The most effective program is to remove all of the cancer before it has spread. This illusory challenge must be equated against the possibility of cure, recognized surgical hazards, surgical mutilation, and possible amelioration against the neoplastic process. There are no prophets, and rarely profits, in this enterprise. It is a potpourri of threat, fear, and possible annihilation, mixed with hope for cure, palliation, and a meaningful life. There is no limit to the trials, experiments, protocols, therapeutic programs, philosophies, calculations, emotions, and fantasies the doctor and the patient can have regarding this confrontation.

By ethics and by law, only the patient can make the decision as to what and how he wishes to be treated. This is supported by his physician and family, second opinions, multiple scientific tests and his own instincts. Under the guise of "informed consent" he makes his decision. There are obvious other techniques of decision making available and practiced, but our democratic mores place the total responsibility upon the person who has the cancer. This burden often approaches the limits of human adaptation. These profound psychic scars are recognized by the surgeon, but have never been adequately addressed. This is how a decision is made regarding one's life or death, one's mutilation, the diminution of one's normative human-ness. It places the burden of pain, disfigurement, loss of physiological function and possible death upon the person who already has the burden of cancer, and then asks that person to make a rational decision concerning his management on the basis of his rights and his autonomy. In one sense, it sounds cruel, but can you propose a better plan?

With this background, my topic for discussion here attains the irrelevant focus of quibbling. The disease speaks for itself, and ultimately is the final decisional determinant. The surgeon's primary responsibility is, first, to attempt to eliminate or diminish the deprivations that are an intimate part of the advance of the cancer. This type of surgical intervention is often a heroic effort that substitutes deformity and disability for the cancer. Most patients gratefully accept this trade-off even though they are regionally crippled and deformed. For the surgeon to superimpose his "ego structure" against this basic premise is presumptuous and tainted with hubris. An honest appraisal of the facts and the consequences of these facts will often suffice to establish the limits of acceptable surgical ablation for the patient and the surgeon. Fundamentally, it is a balance between abnormal speech, breathing, swallowing, mucous, and appearance and a chance for survival or palliation.

Patients, the public, and the medical profession abhor mutilation in any form, and this acts as a general deterrent to excessively mutilating surgical procedures. On the other hand, few surgeons will substitute an inadequate operation for cancer if they feel there is a real chance for cure. Unfortunately, many of their well-planned procedures *prove* to be inadequate, necessitating additional modalities of treatment.

There are rare instances, in the area of the head and neck, where a purely palliative operation may be performed. The criteria of assuming it will not make the patient more uncomfortable, that it will reduce pain, ulceration, bleeding and foulness, and improve the quality of life for a short interval place severe restrictions upon its clinical application.

Many of the operations that are planned for therapeutic cure prove to be only palliations in the end. These major surgical techniques are, however, now routinely combined with postoperative radiotherapy, and palliation is accomplished in certain instances by altering the method of dying. It is much easier for the patient to die of distant metastasis than of uncontrolled cancer at the primary site. When a decision has been made that the primary cancer is not curable, the surgeon must opt for gross subtotal resection with postoperative irradiation, or irradiation and chemotherapy alone, as palliative instruments. Some of these palliative programs can be delivered without serious down-grading of the patient's status for a short period of time. In certain instances, palliative measures cause severe deprivation of normative living standards.

It is now apparent that there is no perfect solution to the treatment of cancer in the head and neck. Regardless of the nuances in the modality of management, the patient must pay a price for his options in therapy and the trade-off in the applications of this therapy. The basic principle of cure remains the highest ethic within the framework of the patient's rights and the skills of the surgeon. The profound biological threat of extensive cancer in this area introduces unpredictable variables that frustrate even the best organized and most hopeful programs. The patient and the surgeon then become locked into a no-win situation where words and theories give way to the pragmatism of temporary survival.

One must have a moralistic posture for treatment. The right program for one person is not necessarily the right program for all persons. The vulnerability of all programs is that the surgeon cannot command the cancer how to behave, and his attempts at controlling it may constitute a series of failures. Adequate treatment at the beginning offers the best chance of cure. To expect to attain this without a deficit of some degree is an illusion. The principle of palliation, in essence, is a planned retreat from life, hoping to get the best out of the dying process by administering an appeasement when this is reasonable.

10

PSYCHOLOGICAL ASPECTS OF MASTECTOMY AND BREAST RECONSTRUCTION AFTER MASTECTOMY

MARY H. McGRATH AND LAURIE A. STEVENS

The emotional chaos that can attend the mastectomy experience has a dual origin: anxiety about cancer and death, and distress at the mutilation of breast amputation. In our society attitudes toward cancer are universally negative with the spectres of a lingering and painful death, dependency for physical care and financial support, and loss of control and self-determination. Facing an uncertain future, there is the fear of an inexorably downhill course despite acquiescence to heroic but dreaded treatments such as ablative surgery, radiotherapy, and chemotherapy.

With mastectomy, the threat to life is accompanied by the emotionally charged dimension of breast loss. An examination of this reaction raises the question of why this body part—the breast—is so important in the individual and collective human experience. The breast is an easily recognized indicator of gender and the exclusive and persistent physical attribute of the female. In addition to physically characterizing femininity, the breast also defines the behavioral role of a woman. Breasts are associated with the uniquely female role of mother and are functionally and symbolically related to the nurturing aspects of motherhood and deep-seated maternal feeling. As a source of sensual and erotic pleasure, breasts are an integral part of female sexuality and as a sexual stimulant to the male, they are an intrinsic feature of female sexual attractiveness. In the context of a woman's total personality, the breast is valued as the symbol of her internalized feelings of femininity, motherliness, and sexuality.

While any woman coming to the mastectomy experience brings her own unique set of attitudes about her sexuality, sexual functioning, and her worth as a person, all experience it to some degree as a degenderizing and dehumanizing event. The loss of a body part is viewed as creating a spoiled or discounted identity. When the body part is sexually relevant, there is a very real threat to the expression of sexuality both in terms of stimulation and responsiveness. Finally, when the body part is implicitly equated with concepts of femininity and inner worth, the mutilation can become emotionally devastating.

PSYCHOLOGICAL REACTIONS TO MASTECTOMY

From an extensive literature, the six most common psychological sequelae of mastectomy are: alterations in mood, characterized by a depressive reaction and lowered self-esteem; alterations in body image, characterized by a diminished sense of wholeness and a sense of asymmetry and body deformity; changes in sexuality, with a diminished feeling of sexual attractiveness and desirability; in femininity, with a notion of feeling and being viewed as less feminine; in social and occupational functioning accompanied by feelings of embarrassment and some inhibition of normal activities; and invariably, a fear of recurrence or spread of the cancer or the development of cancer in the opposite breast (Asken 1975; Clifford 1979; Jamison, Wellisch, and Pasnau 1978; Rennecker and Cutler 1952). The magnitude and generalization of these sequelae are documented in a number of studies.

Roberts and his associates (1972) described a report of depression or anxiety in 51 percent of their sample of women who had had mastectomy. Similarly, in a group of 14 postmastectomy patients, Jamison, Wellisch, and Pasnau 1978) found an increase in suicidal death (24.4 percent), sleep difficulties (9.8 percent), tranquilizer use (35.9 percent), and a decrease in appetite (7.3 percent) and sexual interest (2.7 percent)—all suggestive of a depressive reaction. Maguire (1976) described the impressively high number of women who reported depressive reactions of varying intensity postmastectomy—83 percent. In this group, 30 percent of the women interviewed three to four months postmastectomy still experienced moderate to marked depression. Twenty-five percent of his patients felt that their sexual relations were affected by the mastectomy, characterized by lessening of sexual desire and enjoyment.

In many of the studies, the predominant psychological reaction to mastectomy is a sense of mutilation and a diminution in feelings of femininity. Renneker and Cutler (1952) recognized the early admixture of the threat to femininity with the fear of cancer and death, and Katz et al. (1970) echoed the impression that the first emotional trauma was related to the implications of the loss of the breast itself. Polivy (1977) agreed that an initial psychological reaction to mastectomy was the sense of endangered femininity. Bard (1972) cited profound feelings of self-rejection and loss of self-esteem, and he felt that early depression soon was accompanied by a phase of self-pity and guilt. A distortion of the self-image due to feelings of deformity, worthlessness, and shame was cited also by Klein (1971).

The process of coming to terms with the loss of a breast is similar to the mourning for the loss of a loved one. The grieving process includes stages of denial, anger, despair, and hopefully eventual acceptance. Goin and Goin (1981) also described another stage called "pseudoacceptance" in which the woman does not seem to experience the anger-depression phase. These women seem to use only massive denial as a defense mechanism to protect themselves from their true feelings. Polivy's study (1977) supports the woman's use of denial to protect herself against the large psychological impact of the mastectomy, and this finding has been further supported by the work of Bard and Waxenberg (1959) and Clifford (1979a). The women who state they have never looked at their mastectomy scar, and the 30 percent (Weinstein, Vetter, and Serensen, 1970) to 50 percent (Jamison, Wellisch, and Pasnau, 1978) reported incidence of "sensations" in a phantom breast are believed to be examples of this unconscious denial.

The very existence of a mourning cycle underlines the significance of the anxiety associated with body deformation compared with the anxiety associated with cancer. Maguire (1976) noted that prior to mastectomy distress was more often related to fears about the cancer and its implications than to breast loss. Following mastectomy, however, the percentage of patients attributing their distress to loss of the breast doubled as these women dealt with the crisis of changing their symmetrical image of themselves to an unbalanced one. Citing their deformity as the main or a significant reason for their depression, these women tended to avoid looking at themselves and to hide their disfigurement from their husbands. Wellisch and co-investigators (1978) noted this pattern of behavior when they reported the startling statistic that nearly two years after mastectomy only 80 percent of husbands had seen their wives unclothed. Mourning the lost breast occurs in patients of all ages and while earlier studies had suggested that mastectomy is smoother for the postmenopausal woman, Goin and Goin (1981) have argued that the older woman may experience the same sense of loss as does the younger patient since the symbolic significance of the breast does not decrease with age.

All of the research on the mastectomy experience indicates that the psychological reactions to mastectomy may endure over lengthy periods of time, but that the vast majority of women eventually cope effectively. Long-range studies have shown that most women resume their preoperative responsibilities and do not show an increased psychosocial disability (Craig, Comstock, and Geiser 1974). However, social habits are altered in up to one-third of patients, expressed mainly in the style of dress and the avoidance of recreational activities such as swimming (Buls et al. 1976).

BREAST RECONSTRUCTION

This then brings us to the women seeking breast reconstruction and her motivations and expectations. A reconstructed breast has no physical function: at best there is diminished sensibility, absent contractility, and absent erotic sensation. Unable to restore function, a surgery-shaped imitation breast is little more than a space occupying mass—as is an external prosthesis. Yet women are presenting in ever-increasing numbers for breast reconstruction and in the last few years there has been such a remarkable increase in the amount of information about reconstruction available in the lay press that it is hard to conceive that there are any women left in the United States who are not at least peripherally aware that a breast can be rebuilt after cancer surgery. Most often it is the woman herself who initiates the search for reconstruction. A study from Duke University Medical Center showed that in contrast to the mastectomy experience, in which there is extensive contact with the health-care system, most patients seeking reconstruction seek the surgery by themselves (Clifford 1979a). In their survey of 65 patients, only 28 percent were informed about the availability of reconstruction by their physicians; the remainder learned about the availability of the procedure from newspaper articles or friends.

Clearly, there is some drive of sufficient strength to motivate these women to undergo an elective surgical procedure to replace a nonfunctional part. Psychological studies of these patients are still in their infancy, but it is only logical that the first question raised was whether these women represented adaptive failures, that is, people who lacked the inner resources to cope with their postmastectomy status. First proposed in 1971 (Goldsmith and Alday), this view that psychologically impoverished women from the "nonacceptance" group were most likely to request breast reconstruction does not appear to be withstanding closer scrutiny. On the contrary, the women appear to be reality-oriented and responding to a drive for restitution and a desire for a body part to be reincorporated into their body concept (Clifford 1979). It is surprising initially to realize that very few women undergo breast reconstruction for secondary gain; meaning, an improved marriage or a changed life-style. Many women have difficulty articulating why they seek reconstruction and they will usually cite the realistic problems associated with clothing selection or the discomfort of prosthetic devices. Then most will tentatively indicate that they feel incomplete, unsure, or unbalanced without a breast and that they wish to restore the sense of being whole, or being normal, or being like themselves again. This theme of restitution and a potentially positive psychological response is evident particularly when these women almost invariably volunteer that they are "doing it for themselves."

PSYCHOLOGICAL REACTIONS
TO BREAST RECONSTRUCTION

If restitution of a self-concept is the primary motivation for seeking breast reconstruction, then the success of an actual operation revolves almost completely around whether this psychological requirement is met. Clifford's (1979) study of 65 women undergoing reconstruction an average of 5.4 years after mastectomy revealed that 55 percent expressed dissatisfaction with their body contour and with themselves as a person. Thirty-two percent indicated that their self-concept as individuals had been affected and that their own view of their femininity, or an inner sense of femininity, rather than the views of others about their femaleness, had changed. Thirty-eight percent had lessened sexual activity, 17 percent were depressed and/or angry, and 26 percent tended to deny, avoid or suppress any mention of cancer. In open-ended psychological interviews, fully 70 percent of the women stated that restoration to a sense of wholeness or normalcy was their primary motivation for surgery. After reconstruction, 80 percent of the women described an improvement in their self-concept, their feelings about their appearance, less self-consciousness in public, and satisfaction with the surgical result. This study also provided an interesting anecdote: four of the 65 patients had a simultaneous mastectomy and reconstruction. None of the usual negative psychological sequelae associated with mastectomy were reported by these women and the researchers noted this remarkable finding.

The question of the timing of breast reconstruction had arisen before and it was widely, if informally, held that a woman undergoing immediate breast reconstruction would be less satisfied with the surgical result than would a woman who had had experience with the mastectomy defect. In 1982, Noone and his collaborators (1982) challenged this view performing immediate reconstruction in a selected group of 30 patients. Using retrospective, postoperative interviews they found a high level of satisfaction with the cosmetic result in patients who were well prepared for mastectomy and immediate reconstruction. Later in 1982, Goin and Goin studied the effect of immediate reconstruction at the time of prophylactic mastectomy in a group of 10 women who had already had a mastectomy for cancer and delayed reconstruction on the opposite side. The women in their study all expressed the wish that immediate reconstruction could have been done at the time of the initial mastectomy.

PSYCHOLOGICAL REACTIONS TO THE TIMING OF BREAST RECONSTRUCTION

As these reports of a favorable patient acceptance of immediate reconstruction were coming to light, we had been observing our patients undergoing simultaneous mastectomy and reconstruction and had developed the impression that whole-life attitudinal differences were present in these women compared with those presenting for delayed reconstruction. A study was organized to examine systematically the short and longer term psychological functioning of patients having immediate breast reconstruction relative to the well described reactions seen after mastectomy. Questions to be answered included whether the process of mourning the lost breast would be altered, impeded, or even aborted by immediate reconstruction. Or would it merely be delayed, and the patient required to come to terms with her loss at a later date? If postmastectomy depression was diminished, how would the psychological benefits of immediate reconstruction compare with those of delayed reconstruction? Lastly, would the woman's attitude toward the reconstructed breast be influenced by the timing of reconstruction? (Stevens et al. 1984).

The study included 13 women who chose immediate reconstruction and 12 women who chose delayed reconstruction anywhere from 3 months to 8 years post-mastectomy. The patients who had immediate reconstruction had an open-ended, semi-structured interview with a psychiatrist immediately after surgery and then at 3 and 6 month intervals. The delayed reconstruction patients were interviewed within 3 months postoperatively. All patients completed a Breast Reconstruction Index questionnaire and a symptom checklist 3 months postoperatively.

PREOPERATIVE CONCERNS

The patients who chose immediate reconstruction admitted to more concerns about the effect of the mastectomy on their feelings of femininity, sexuality, and their body symmetry than did those who chose delayed reconstruction. This group seemed to invest equal importance in the feeling that they would be "deformed" as on the cancer itself. They felt that the mastectomy would rid them of the cancer and the reconstruction would repair the damage done by the mastectomy.

POSTOPERATIVE CONCERNS—DEPRESSION

The group who underwent immediate reconstruction reported fewer depressive symptoms than did the delayed reconstruction group (23 percent versus 83 percent), postmastectomy. The delayed reconstruction group reported an improvement in mood and a diminution in depressive symptoms after reconstruction. There was some difference in the report of a feeling of loss for the breast in the two groups: 100 percent in the delayed reconstruction and 69 percent in the immediate reconstruction group. The three patients in the latter group who denied feelings of loss seemed to be using denial as their primary coping mechanism. These women denied any significant impact of the surgery on their lives or feelings about themselves or their bodies. There was a similar set of 4 patients in the delayed reconstruction group who, although reporting feelings of loss, denied an impact of the mastectomy before reconstruction on their lives or their feelings; yet they sought reconstruction. The women who described feelings of loss also described a mourning for the lost breast which included feelings of sadness and anger. This mourning process seemed to begin even before the surgery with the anticipated loss of the breast. The timing of breast reconstruction did not appear to alter substantially the mourning process.

POSTOPERATIVE CONCERNS—BODY IMAGE

Body image disturbance was a large concern for both groups, the immediate reconstruction group preoperatively and for the delayed group, postmastectomy. Seventy-five percent of the delayed group reported feeling "deformed" after mastectomy while none of the immediate group had such feelings. All of those who had felt deformed described the reconstruction as repairing those feelings. It was noteworthy that several of these women explained that the knowledge of a potential reconstruction had helped to minimize the negative impact of the mastectomy on their body image; they appeared to have used a fantasy of the reconstructed breast to aid their psychological adjustment. Of the immediate reconstruction group, 92 percent described their reconstruction as "restoration" of the lost breast and 8 percent (one patient) described it as "replacement." Of the delayed group, only 25 percent regarded the reconstruction as "restoration" while the majority expressed the concept of "replacement."

All of the delayed reconstruction group felt that the external prosthesis that they wore after mastectomy was a burden and a discomfort and none experienced the prosthesis as either a restoration or a replacement of the breast. Fifty percent had altered their clothing after mastectomy, wearing looser clothing in an effort to draw attention away from their breasts. They all regarded the reconstructed breast as a liberating experience, permitting a return to their premastectomy style of clothing and activity. None of the immediate group changed their style of dress.

POSTOPERATIVE CONCERNS—SEXUALITY AND FEMININITY

Only one patient (8 percent) in the immediate group felt that her sexual attractiveness was diminished and this patient was receiving chemotherapy, but the others reported a return to their preoperative sexual functioning. The level of return to sexual functioning seemed to correspond with a feeling of sexual attractiveness because 58 percent of the delayed group experienced a diminution of both after mastectomy, and 75 percent reported feeling enhanced attractiveness and improvement in sexual functioning after reconstruction.

POSTOPERATIVE CONCERNS—OTHER

There did not seem to be any significant difference between the two groups in the timing of return to occupational or social functioning.

In both groups, the patients who were most concerned about tumor recurrence were those receiving chemotherapy for microscopic spread to the axillary lymph nodes. The timing of reconstruction did not alter the cancer concerns.

There was a striking difference between the two groups in their knowledgeability about breast cancer—the women in the immediate group seemed to be more inquisitive and participated in all stages of the decision making regarding their cancer and their surgery. They had considered alternative treatments for their breast cancer, including radiotherapy, lumpectomy with axillary dissection, mastectomy alone, and delayed and immediate reconstruction. Most of the delayed group denied having learned about alternative treatments. When questioned about whether they would have immediate reconstruction if cancer returned in the opposite breast, all of the immediate group and 11/12 of the delayed group responded affirmatively.

POSTOPERATIVE CONCERNS—
SATISFACTION WITH THE SURGICAL RESULT

All of the delayed reconstruction group were satisfied with their cosmetic results stating it was equivalent to their expectations. Two of the 13 women in the immediate group stated the result far exceeded expectations, but one was not fully satisfied. When her dissatisfaction was explored, she revealed that she had always wished her breasts were larger and had anticipated the reconstruction would produce a larger sized breast and that she then would have had a good reason to seek augmentation on the opposite side. It was this patient who was the one in the immediate group who felt the breast reconstruction was just a replacement for the missing breast and not a restoration. Several of the patients have sought a reduction mammaplasty or a mastopexy for their remaining healthy breast to further body symmetry and all of the women have had or are planning nipple-areolar reconstruction. The whole issue of symmetry seems to have special importance.

PHYSICIAN–PATIENT RELATIONSHIP

All of the patients remarked that they welcomed the opportunity to meet with a psychiatrist and related the difficulty they had discussing, even with sexual partners and close female friends, their deeper concerns, especially with regard to issues of sexuality and femininity.

SUMMARY OF THE STUDY

This study showed that a great psychological benefit can be derived from simultaneous reconstruction with mastectomy. The improved quality of life postoperatively for these women, compared with the prereconstruction delayed group, is statistically startling. Initial concerns that immediate reconstruction would alter or impede the process of mourning and adaptation were proved unnecessary. The results suggest that grieving for the breast loss begins in both groups even before surgery with the anticipation of the loss.

What had not been anticipated at the outset was there would be any prevailing difference between the immediate group and the other patients after they had finally had reconstruction. The difference in the degree of integration of the breast mound into the body image was unexpected. That the immediate group would experience the surgical result as a restoration rather than a replacement, and that the converse would exist in the delayed group, may be very important to a woman's sense of personal integrity.

The findings emanating from this work should be considered suggestive rather than definitive. The number of patients in the study groups was small and much of the data were retrospective. To enhance the study a third group of patients who had mastectomy alone and did not choose breast reconstruction could be added. The study was not double blind in that the interviewer knew the timing of the patient's reconstructive procedure. A future project might begin with a thorough psychological assessment of the patient's premorbid status, and it would be especially useful to assess the reactions of family and spouses to the surgery since their reactions may have a significant impact on the woman's attitude. There is also the problem that the women who choose immediate breast reconstruction are a self-selected group, and this may bias the findings; however, there does not seem to be any way to eliminate this bias.

CONCLUSIONS

The considerable psychiatric morbidity which may follow mastectomy for breast cancer is caused by anxiety at the knowledge that the patient has cancer and by distress about the mutilation caused by the operation. The relative contribution of each of these factors to the mastectomy experience may vary widely from one woman to another. Certainly their impact cannot be disassociated from the individual's premorbid psychological make-up, the symbolic significance of her breasts, and the very practical consideration of the extent and stage of the cancer.

It is clear, however, that some proportion of the distress with mastectomy is related to the resultant disfigurement and damage to the self-image. Breast reconstruction appears to meet the psychological requirements for restitution and provision of a restored self-concept. Preliminary studies now suggest that the timing of breast reconstruction has a strong impact on the psychological "success" of the operation. Immediate breast reconstruction reduces the negative emotional sequelae of breast loss and appears to do this more effectively than delayed reconstruction. In the surgically suitable woman with early breast cancer, this modality may help to lessen the psychological trauma of the painful experience of breast loss.

REFERENCES

Asken, M.J. 1975. "Psychoemotional Aspects of Mastectomy: A Review of Recent Literature." *American Journal of Psychiatry* 132:56–59.

Bard, M. 1972. "The Sequence of Emotional Reactions in Radical Mastectomy Patients." *Health Report* 67:1144–1148.

Bard, M. and S. Waxenberg. 1959. "Relationship of Cornell Medical Index to Postsurgical Invalidism." *Journal of Clinical Psychology* 13:151–153.

Buls, J.G., I.H. Jones, A.C. Bennett, and D.P. Chan. 1976. "Women's Attitudes to Mastectomy for Breast Cancer." *Austrian Medical Journal* 2:336–338.

Clifford, E. 1979. "Psychological Effects of the Mastectomy Experience." In N.G. Georgiade, ed., *Breast Reconstruction Following Mastectomy*, St. Louis: C.V. Mosby, pp. 1–21.

Clifford, E. 1979a. "The Reconstructive Experience: The Search for Restitution."

In N.G. Georgiade, ed., *Breast Reconstruction Following Mastectomy*, St. Louis: C.V. Mosby, pp. 22–34.

Craig, T.J., G.W. Comstock, and P.B. Geiser. 1974. "The Quality of Survival in Breast Cancer: A Case-Control Comparison." *Cancer* 33:1451–1457.

Goin, J.M. and M.K. Goin. 1981. "Breast Reconstruction After Mastectomy." In *Changing the Body: Psychological Effects of Plastic Surgery.* Baltimore: Williams and Wilkins, pp. 163–169.

Goin, M.K. and J.M. Goin. 1982. "Psychological Reactions to Prophylactic Mastectomy Synchronous with Contralateral Breast Reconstruction." *Plastic and Reconstructive Surgery* 70:355–359.

Goldsmith, H.S. and E.S. Alday. 1971. "Role of the Surgeon in the Rehabilitation of the Breast Cancer Patient." *Cancer* 28:1672–1675.

Jamison, K., D.K. Wellisch, and R.O. Pasnau. 1978. "Psychological Aspects of Mastectomy: I. The Woman's Perspective." *American Journal of Psychiatry* 135:432–436.

Katz, J.L., H. Weiner, T.L. Gallagher, and L. Hellman. 1970. "Stress, Distress and Ego Defenses—Psychoendocrine Responses to Impending Breast Tumor Biopsy." *Archives of General Psychiatry* 23:131–142.

Klein, R.A. 1971. "A Crisis to Grow on." *Cancer* 28:1660–1665.

Maguire, P. 1976. "The Psychological and Social Sequelae of Mastectomy." In J.G. Howells, ed., *Modern Perspectives in the Psychiatric Aspects of Surgery*, New York: Brunner/Mazel Inc., Chapter 19.

Noone, R.B., T.G. Frazier, C.Z. Hayward, and M.S. Skiles. 1982. "Patient Acceptance of Immediate Reconstruction Following Mastectomy." *Plastic and Reconstructive Surgery* 69:632–638.

Polivy, J. 1977. "Psychological Effects of Mastectomy on a Woman's Feminine Self-Concept." *Journal of Nervous and Mental Disorders* 164:77–87.

Renneker, R. and M. Cutler. 1952. "Psychological Problems of Adjustment to Cancer of the Breast." *Journal of the American Medical Association* 148:833–839.

Roberts, M.D., S.G. Furnival, and A.P.M. Forrest. 1972. "The Morbidity of Mastectomy." *British Journal of Surgery* 59:301–302.

Stevens, L.A., M.H. McGrath, R.G. Druss, S.J. Kister, F.E. Gump, and K.A. Forde. 1984. "The Psychological Impact of Immediate Breast Reconstruction for Women with Early Breast Cancer." *Plastic and Reconstructive Surgery*, 73:619–628.

Weinstein, S., R.J. Vetter, and E.A. Serensen. 1970. "Phantoms Following Breast Amputation." *Neuropsychologia* 8:185–197.

Wellisch, D.K., K.R. Jamison, and R.O. Pasnau. 1978. "Psychosocial Aspects of Mastectomy: II. The Man's Perspective." *American Journal of Psychiatry* 135:543–546.

11

HYSTERECTOMY:
A BRIEF LOOK AT PSYCHOSOCIAL ASPECTS

PHYLLIS C. LEPPERT

In terms of physical appearance the removal of the uterus is not mutilating surgery. Vaginal hysterectomy leaves no noticeable scar and abdominal hysterectomy can be accomplished in such a manner as to leave a barely noted residual scar near the pubic hair line. Therefore, the fact that a woman has undergone surgery for the removal of the uterus is known only to the woman herself and to those close to her. Hysterectomies are done for various indications—benign as well as malignant. Most commonly they are done for curative purposes and are not life-threatening. In spite of this, a hysterectomy is life-altering. No matter how sophisticated or educated the individual woman is the loss of the womb and the ability to bear children necessitates reorganization of her perception of herself. The reasons are deep-seated and have their origins in childhood experiences, past parental attitudes and perceptions, present expectations and current relationships with others, both men and women. All are modulated by cultural attitudes. More than any other part of a woman's body, the uterus represents what is perceived as the essence of womanhood. Having a uterus sets a woman apart.

Most women have superimposed on this subconscious, often magical perception of hysterectomy, other concerns and expectations that they have adopted through education and continuing changes in cultural roles. As society has placed less emphasis on motherhood and more on women's intellectual and productive skills, a hysterectomy is less traumatic than it was in the past. Advances in reproductive science and

73

biology have allowed the gynecologist to treat more women successfully with conservative treatment, and therefore accepted surgical indications for hysterectomy are narrower now than in the earlier decades of this century (Thompson 1981). Gynecological practice has changed so that it is possible to carry out conservative surgery for malignant disease occurring in the childbearing years, for instance, and doing the definitive surgery—hysterectomy—later after the desired pregnancies. Early accurate diagnosis aided by ultrasound and hormonal radioimmunoassays combined with aggressive drug therapy for pelvic inflammatory disease and endometriosis has contributed to a drastic reduction in the indications for hysterectomy. Since women in the United States today have fewer pregnancies than women during the early decades of this century and, in general, are very aware of health and fitness, uterine prolapse and descensus is decreasing as a reason for the removal of the uterus. Women also desire more second opinions now, and this may be another important fact in the decreasing indications for hysterectomy (Thompson 1981).

Despite this trend, in the United States, 3,536,000 women in the reproductive years underwent hysterectomies from 1970 to 1978 (Center for Disease Control 1981; Dicker et al. 1982). There are wide regional practices regarding this surgery. There were more hysterectomies performed in the South as opposed to the Northeast. More vaginal hysterectomies as opposed to abdominal hysterectomies were done in the West. However, more women in the Northeast had their ovaries and tubes removed along with their uterus (Dicker et al. 1982). It is not known if these regional differences reflect contrasts in the severity of disease.

Studies of the emotional reactions of women to hysterectomy are virtually nonexistent. There are reports of psychiatric symptoms, such as depression or referral to psychiatric care following this surgery (Barker 1968). Other studies offer conflicting evidence and indicate that there is no real increase in psychological sequelae after hysterectomy (Mills 1973; Hampton and Tarnasky 1974; Gath, Cooper, and Day 1982; Gath et al. 1982). Other researchers point to the fact that women appear to have high levels of preoperative psychiatric morbidity which confounds the reported postoperative findings (Gath, Cooper, and Day 1982; Martin, Roberts, and Clayton 1980). Many of the reported studies are confounded by mixed gynecological indications for hysterectomy. In addition, little preoperative evaluation is done and there is a poor definition of psychiatric morbidity.

The two studies by Gath et al. were well designed and included the administration of pre and postoperative standardized psychological tests. They discovered that the psychological outcome after hysterectomy was strongly associated with preoperative mental state, neuroticism, previous psychiatric history, and family psychiatric history but *not* with gynecological pathology, age, parity, marital status, or socioeconomic class. Interestingly, the subject's psychiatric symptoms were lessened after hysterectomy, which in this study was done for benign disease with significant symptoms.

In terms of understanding the emotional impact of hysterectomy these studies do not really help. They do tell us that some women in some situations cannot cope effectively with the stress that this surgery brings to their lives. These studies do not mean that women do not have emotional reactions to and adjustments to make regarding hysterectomy. They do mean that many women *cope* with the stress of the removal of their uterus without the development of overt psychiatric symptoms. Health care professionals must learn to help women undergoing this surgery in understanding their emotions and in adjusting to them.

What then are some of the emotional reactions women have to hysterectomy? These will be individual, and clinicians need to listen carefully to each patient. Consciously expressed emotions may mask underlying feelings. In general, the emotional responses will vary not only from woman to woman but within each individual. A premenopausal woman with teenage children may be glad to be finished with menstruation, but be sad that her youth is over. One married woman, for example, who had not had children needed a hysterectomy in her late forties. She expressed the opinion that her uterus had not done her any good anyway so she might as well be rid of it. A newly arrived woman from the west coast of Africa said she would rather die than have a hysterectomy and she meant it literally. In her culture, a woman unable to have children would be rejected by her husband and divorced without question. The value a society places on women in other aspects of life besides motherhood has a role to play in how women within that society will react to hysterectomy. How the woman copes with and grieves for her loss of childbearing potential is inherent in her personality and ego strength as well as the support she receives from other persons.

If the hysterectomy is done for advanced malignancy the woman will have two stresses; that of facing a life-threatening disease and that of the surgery itself. It is important to realize that depression or grief expressed in this case may be due to anxieties about the nature of the disease itself and not to the hysterectomy.

Although age made no difference in prevalence of psychiatric disturbance after hysterectomy, a single woman of reproductive years will undoubtedly view a hysterectomy as drastically altering her life options. All women fear that a hysterectomy will alter their sexuality. Some think that they will not be able to function and have intercourse; some feel that they will not be seen as desirable sexual objects. Some of these fears can be based on facts. If the ovaries are removed along with the uterus the vagina may lose its pliability and may not lubricate well. Without a contracting uterus at orgasm some pleasurable sensations maybe lost. Since men are subjected to many deeply rooted emotions also, they may have magical notions about the uterus and subconsciously reject a woman who has had a hysterectomy. On a positive side, both men and women may be relieved that birth control is no longer necessary.

A sensitive clinician must appreciate that all women will have emotional reactions to hysterectomy and that coping behaviors will vary. Women will adjust to this stress as they have to other stresses in their lives. In treating women who undergo hysterectomies as individuals and in giving them time to talk, to feel their emotions; in giving them concerned support and explanations underlying the treatment of their diseases, physicians can help each woman maximize her adjustment to the surgery.

REFERENCES

Barker, M.G. 1968. "Psychiatric Illness After Hysterectomy." *British Medical Journal* 1:91–95.

Center for Disease Control. 1981. "Hysterectomy in Women Age 15–44 in U.S. 1970–78." *Connecticut Medicine* 45:663–664.

Dicker, R.C., M.J. Scally, J.R. Greenspan, P.M. Loyde, H.W. Ory, J.M. Maze, and J.C. Smith. 1982. "Hysterectomies Among Women of Reproductive Age." *Journal of the American Medical Association* 248:323–327.

Gath, D., P. Cooper, A. Bond, and G. Edmonds. 1982. "Hysterectomy and Psychiatric Disorders. II. Demographic, Psychiatric and Physical Factors in Relation to Psychiatric Outcome." *British Journal of Psychiatry* 140:343–350.

Gath, D., P. Cooper, and A. Day. 1982. "Hysterectomy and Psychiatric Disorder. I. Levels of Psychiatric Morbidity Before and After Hysterectomy." *British Journal of Psychiatry* 140:335–342.

Hampton, P.T. and W.G. Tarnasky. 1974. "Hysterectomy and Tubal Ligation: A

Comparison of the Psychological Aftermath." *American Journal of Obstetrics and Gynecology* 119:949–952.

Martin, R.L., W.V. Roberts, and P.J. Clayton. 1970. "Psychiatric Status After Hysterectomy — A One Year Prospective Follow-up." *Journal of the American Medical Association* 244:350–353.

Mills, W.G. 1973. "Depression After Hysterectomy." *Lancet* II:672.

Singh, B., et al. 1983. "Post-hysterectomy Adaptation: A Review and Report of Two Follow-up Studies." *Australia-New Zealand Journal of Psychiatry* 17:

Thompson, J.D. 1981. "Indications for Hysterectomy." *Clinical Obstetrics and Gynecology* 24:1245–1258.

12

OSTOMIES

ROBERT G. BERTSCH

Abdominal stomas can create several problems in the lives of people who must have them. It is estimated that each year in this country 100,000 new gastrointestinal or urinary stomas are created and 16,000 are closed. Thus, 84,000 new stomas are added annually. What kinds of people are involved? The great majority of patients with permanent abdominal ostomies fall into three categories: patients with inflammatory bowel disease, colorectal cancer, or cystectomized patients in need of urinary diversion. The first group tends to be younger; the cancer patients tend to be older; the conduit patients are often children. Thus, all socioeconomic and age groups in the United States are involved.

The stoma itself should not create a disability. Physically, a healthy, well-cared for stoma is comfortable, painless, and does not interfere with physical activity of any kind. Equipment worn over it is lightweight and inconspicuous under normal fashionable clothing. However, many patients do not perceive their stomas in this way.

The conditions and diseases being treated may introduce other problems that prevent the patient from functioning normally even though the stoma is perfect. In addition, the patients are often faced with additional surgery related to the stomas, especially in the early years following the original operation. These repeats can be the result of staged operations, the result of continued disease, and later on even the need for revision.

Emotionally, a stoma is a difficult change for most patient to accept. The first handicap an ostomy patient is faced with is that society has not accepted having the excretory orifices removed from their God-given site. Ostomies are not a subject one talks about in polite society. As a taboo subject, ostomies are perceived as a handicap.

The second handicap presented by an ostomy is the difficulty in obtaining specialized medical care. Too many inexperienced surgeons perform these operations. Stomas are placed in unusable locations or are incorrectly formed. Not enough hospitals use enterostomal therapists to properly educate these patients preoperatively and postoperatively.

Insurance companies often reject ostomy patients, causing them great difficulty in obtaining health, hospital, and life insurance, a third handicap.

A fourth handicap is vocational. Patients who return to work may find simple things like bathroom privacy not available. Patients often do not return to their original jobs, and older patients approaching retirement age often retire early using their stoma as an excuse.

Fifth, there is difficulty in selecting and using the numerous prostheses available. The know-how is intricate and varied for each special situation. Improper choice and/or use of equipment leads to soiling, skin breakdown, and odor—all of which quickly force the patient to stay home in isolation.

The greatest handicap of all is a shortage of rehabilitation programs for ostomy patients. These are sorely needed in hospitals and in outpatient clinics. As the rehabilitation period is under way, ostomy patients and their families must get information that is accurate, helpful, and understandable. The concern of the patient is appliance function, trustworthiness of equipment, and expense of equipment (often not covered by health insurance). All patients worry about the stoma: can it be damaged; what about bleeding, size change, skin trouble, gas, and odor, what foods should be avoided? Patient education before surgery, as a combined effort of the surgeon, enterostomal therapist, and nursing staff and perhaps by a person who has experienced this operation, seems to be the most important factor in rehabilitation.

Also, there are always worries about recurrence of disease which is especially important in the cancer and Crohn's disease patients.

Sexual power is of special concern to many of these patients. Attitudes toward sexuality should be considered in three ways: the stoma itself, the attitude toward the stoma, and the physical impairment of function as a result of the surgery. The stoma is considered delicate and destroyable by the average patient and/or spouse. It is difficult to convince a couple that this should in no way affect their intimacy and close contact. The attitude toward the stoma can be a serious problem. However, in the final analysis if a couple has a close and fulfilling relation before the surgery, it is most often continued after. The major sexual problems occur in relationships that were shaky to begin with.

Physical dysfunction caused by the surgery itself (impotence in males and dyspareunia in females) is the most serious and difficult problem to correct. This is more common in cancer patients as opposed to patients with inflammatory bowel disease.

Although colostomies have been made since the turn of the century, ileostomies and conduits are relatively newer procedures, being first performed in the 1940s and 1950s respectively. Numerous improvements for ostomy patients in this period have contributed to the acceptance of these operations.

First and foremost, with the development of new stapling devices, surgeons are having to do fewer permanent colostomies in cases of rectal and low-lying rectosigmoid cancers. If ostomies have to be performed, the newer appliances worn over stomas are lighter, easier to use, more protective of the periostomal skin, and cheaper than earlier devices. Something should be said about the Kock pouch, a procedure obviating the need for an appliance. This is a continent ileostomy performed after total colectomy. Finally, with the development of the enterostomal therapists training program, hospitals are able to provide experts to help ostomy patients function more normally. Most major hospitals are making use of graduates of this program.

Although these improvements are of significant help to the ostomy patient in functioning in a normal manner, we must help the patient cope with the loss of a part and the associated loss of self-image when it affects sexuality. We must help patients deal with the fear of recurrence in cases of Crohn's disease or cancer. Educational counseling, especially preoperatively when possible but certainly postoperatively and in the follow-up period, is the most important item for a successful rehabilitation of the ostomy patient. The surgeon, nurse, and enterostomal therapist comprise a multidisciplinary team that must be available to these patients.

PART IV
INTERDISCIPLINARY CARE
AND DISCLOSURE OF INCURABILITY

13

PURVEYORS OF CONTINUING CARE
FOR THE INCURABLE PATIENT

JAY I. MELTZER

I am disturbed by the use of the term purveyor. I don't think of myself, and I hope patients don't think of me, as a purveyor. I have been and will continue to be a doctor for dying patients who want one and, I hope, in the way they want one. Purvey has a pejorative tone, implying merchandizing, whereas the heart of doctoring is beneficence, even though fee is exchange for service. To use the word purvey suggests a one-sided provider, paternalistic orientation, whereas doctors basically and truly respond to human needs. These needs are properly demands because they are based in the right to medical care. Patients need to be less timid and more forthright in clearly stating their demands, not in general, but in specific medical situations, face-to-face with doctors. This fosters dialogue, information exchange, the essential element in all medical care that respects patient autonomy.

Does the role of doctor to incurable dying patients differ from other doctoring roles? Once all are agreed the situation is hopeless, does that change things? Is the doctor made inadequate, less necessary or ineffective? Should care be turned over, or partly delegated, to others? If so, who is "in charge?"

Doctoring means dealing with the twin problems of symptoms and suffering. Symptoms are the felt consequences of disease for the body: pain. Suffering is the impact of disease on a life, a particular predicament, concerning one's hopes, family, loved ones, and job. Doctoring is no different with the dying. There are still symptoms and suffering to be relieved right up to the end.

So much for theory. The practice of medicine is empirical. It evolves from experience and tradition, passed on from one doctoral generation to another, continually modified by current scientific concepts. The practice of medicine is also moral. The moral precepts are also passed on, changed, modified by current values. It is interesting to note what changes and what stays the same.

When I began practice in 1958, most physicians were guided by the concept that medical information was to be treated like medication, given in therapeutic doses, completely at the discretion of the physician. There was very little mention of the patient's right to know. Whenever the news was bad, there was usually little one could do about it anyway. Physician-patient dialogue was inhibited by the concept that patients could be physically injured by bad news, and were incapable of accepting, or even comprehending, such news.

The American Medical Association's code of ethics at the time, in the section describing the duties of physicians to their patients, said:

> The physician should not fail, on proper occasions, to give the friends of the patient timely notice of danger, when it really occurs; and even to the patient himself, if absolutely necessary. This office, however, is so peculiarly alarming, when executed by the physician that it ought to be declined whenever it can be assigned to any other person of sufficient judgment and delicacy. For the physician should be the minister of hope and comfort to the sick, that by such cordials to the drooping spirit, he may smooth the bed of death, revive expiring life, and counteract the depressing influence of those maladies which often disturb the tranquility of the most resigned, in their last moments. The life of a sick person can be shortened not only by the acts, but also the words or the manner of a physician.

The code went on to state that the physician should not abandon the incurable, "for his attendance can be highly useful to the patient, and comforting to the relatives around him, even in the last period of a fatal malady, by alleviating pain and other symptoms, and by soothing mental anguish." To decline attendance would be to "sacrifice moral duty to fanciful delicacy."

Once in practice, I remember the struggle my fellow internists had with this dual injunction. Do not abandon the incurable, but at the same time, do not give any bad news, and be careful not to injure by acts or manner. Quite an order! Internists solved the problem the only way it could be solved, by ingenious lying. Lying was often just that. But there were those who, uncomfortable with outright lies, devel-

oped imaginative ways of truth telling that patients would not comprehend unless they were extraordinarily clear-headed and determined
to get the truth. Sharing practice at the start with older internists,
I recall a case of a patient operated on for abdominal cancer and
found to have liver metastases. This person was told the diagnosis
was hepatitis. Indeed, cancerous infiltration of the liver does produce
a sort of hepatitis. Next came the insinuation this was good news,
readily accepted by the patient whose unspoken preoperative fear was
cancer in the first place. Next came the explanation that the course
of hepatitis was unpredictable, variable, complicated, likely to get worse
before it got better, setting the stage for any future event. This myth
would last to the end. The family was told the truth. The family usually
had the firm belief that the patient not be told the truth, so there
was rarely conflict with prevailing medical practice. Lest we judge this
apparent conspiracy too harshly by today's standards, let me stress that
the doctor then stayed to the end. That meant setting up home care with
whatever was needed: proper equipment; beds, commodes, walkers,
suction, oxygen, mattresses, proper personnel; nurses, aides, technicians,
and the conflicts they brought to the home, and, of course, proper
attending; house visits, and telephone access. This access to the many
little questions that come up in the care of the homebound, or even
hospitalized, terminally ill, is indispensable to the frightened family
living in or out. And it had to be 24 hours a day, with coverage on the
weekends off.

Who can provide this kind of care? Who knows how to say to each
person involved, patient and family, it isn't your fault in a way each will
believe enough to be comforted? Only the one who knows all the players:
the internist as family physician. This means attention to details. The
doctors who showed me how to do that transferred something of value,
something that never changes. That some of them misled is not so
important now. That has changed. They created myths that would allow
for attentive and compassionate care to the end. Concerns for our present day belief in the independent value of truthtelling may obscure the
fact that yesterday truthtelling was a lesser good, felt to be in conflict
with compassionate care—the higher goal. No doubt there was secondary gain to this concept. The doctor never had to admit or confront cruel
facts. To that extent, the patient never lost confidence in the physician,
which was closely connected to hope. This type of lying also served to

protect the authority of the physician and had value for both patient and family who gained something from that gift.

What has happened to change things?

First, we have been relieved of the belief that most patients cannot take bad news. Telling the truth does not invariably lead to depression, but, in many, improves the quality of the life remaining. Still, the decision to tell the truth or to lie must be made and carried out in a fallible human context.

Second, the increased awareness of patient's rights, patient autonomy, has called attention to the unpleasant aspects of lying. People are entitled to all the information which concerns them, and withholding or distorting it is now seen as subtle coercion and improper use of medical authority.

Third, the increase in the numbers of professionals involved in the delivery of health care, and the increased sense of autonomy that extends not only to patients, but also to nurses, aides, medical students, interns, technicians, social workers and more, has made lying extremely difficult tactically.

Lastly, the major advances of scientific medicine have made the assessment of incurability more complicated. Now when the surgeon finds widespread metastases, it is not just a question of making the patient comfortable, but what is the best way to continue treatment? Such lying or deception as was morally possible in the past has now become extremely difficult. There is no story that will explain away the complicated process of chemotherapy or radiotherapy. The fact of modern cancer therapy is a major reason for truthtelling in inoperable neoplastic disease. Thus, technology changes the moral rules of medicine, forcing us to confront fate and facts. This new technology has also changed the very concept of treatment itself. Cure, or at least return to normal health, was always the goal even if one often had to settle for less. Modern technology has created the concept of palliation, now a goal in itself. This means treatment with no hope of cure. The new goal is not normalcy, but some compromised state preferable to some worse alternative. One can palliate cancer for years at some level approaching normal health, and later on, at successively diminished levels of health. From this a new question arises. When is the situation hopeless? Or should I say, when does one stop treatment? Isn't there always some new, as yet not fully tested, agent to try when the patient has lost ground from the previous level of palliation? Is death the only end of the game? Is there some point when one no longer should fight? If so, who decides? The patient? The doctor? The family? The courts? The Congress? Is it enough to say that if patient and doctor agree, the family or society has no further say? Surely the doctor alone cannot decide for someone else what quality of life is acceptable unless, of course, that someone cannot decide for himself. Who is best qualified to create the proper forum for solution of these complex questions?

In telling my story this way, I am building the case for the internist as the one best qualified to orchestrate the complexities of continuing care for the incurable. The internist has the requisite skills, training and tradition, as well as the infrastructure necessary to meet all the needs of the patient. The internist as family physician knows all the players, is in a position to prepare self and patient by developing the necessary dialogue over many years. In check-ups and in the handling of specific medical problems, large and small, doctor and patient can get practice in exchanging information, in building dialogue.

But, who is "in charge?" Whoever the patient wants to be! What does being "in charge" mean? Whatever a patient, in dialogue with the "in charge person" wants it to mean! Ours is still a demand system respecting patients' needs and rights.

I hope patients will freely choose the internist. I hope internists recognize the importance of this role, and respond when called. Technologic excellence and scientific power should not be allowed to separate us from our humanity. Nowhere is this better practiced than when we admit scientific failure, death, and then stay to the end.

Doctors are not the only ones who can be found short on commitment to compassionate care. Doctors are being targeted and faulted for what may be a generalized diminution in compassion and caring. It is sad, and inexcusable, for a caring family who wants home care for a dying member not to be able to find a compassionate physician to be responsible. It is also troublesome for a doctor to want to give such care and to find no way to give it in the institutional setting of his or her practice. Hopefully, doctors and patients can become allies, make known what is wanted and needed, and clearly demand it of the coming generation before this type of care is regulated, administered, or ignored out of existence.

14

THE RECURRENCE

FREDERICK M. GOLOMB

As a surgeon with over 30 years of experience taking care of patients with cancer, I am still not hardened to the shock and disappointment when a cancer recurs. It means I have failed. It means my patient is quite probably going to die. It means I have a job to do.

As soon as I discover the recurrence, I start thinking about a program of action. This includes not only additional tests, studies, and a plan of therapy, but also how to handle the emotional impact on the patient. In other words, I must prepare myself for the disclosure to the patient.

First, I must break the news. There are as many ways to do this as there are patients. Each patient is unique and each must be handled individually. As an intimate of the patient, the surgeon is in a special position to do the job. The surgeon has lived with the patient through the anxieties and pain of the primary operation and knows the patient's strengths and weaknesses. He has seen him at regular follow-up visits and, as a consequence of this close and sustained relationship, an intimacy develops. A sense of dependency is then built up in the patient; a feeling of continuing responsibility develops in the surgeon. So when the recurrence is recognized, there is a role the surgeon must take that cannot be shrugged off or delegated to anyone else.

As an example, I propose a hypothetical patient, Bob Strong. He came to me with this little mole on his upper thigh. It looked harmless enough to him, but I knew it carried a lethal potential. He was told then that there were statistics that predicted the probability of cure or failure, but I stressed the optimistic side of the ledger. Following the surgery, I saw him at regular intervals. Months went by, then a year and then two passed without trouble. Three years after his operation bumps could be felt under the skin. I knew what they meant, and a dreadful scenario filled my mind. I could foresee and predict the future! Bob's days were numbered. He came up on the wrong side of the ledger. What to do? By now, we were friends and he relied on me. When the biopsy confirmed metastatic melanoma, I had to tell him. "Bob, I have disturbing news for you. The cancer has recurred." Did he hear me? Did he really know the enormity of that statement? Did he realize what lay on the road ahead? Could he possibly know what I know? I had to lead him gently into the picture and stress the positive. "Fortunately, it is localized to the skin and it should respond to therapy."

Would I tell him now of all the rocks and pitfalls that lay ahead in his path—the steadily downhill road to oblivion? Or should I take his hand and meet each hurdle as it came? Questions will come, and I must anticipate them. I must know as much about his disease and its treatment as possible. I must learn who will be best to help him.

"Okay," he said, "when do we start treatment? Who's going to treat me? If you send me to someone else you'll be calling the shots, won't you?"

"Of course," I said, "I'll still be in charge." That reassurance was essential. Although I knew that eventually his day-to-day care would fall into others' hands, it was important that our relationship at this point remain close. Furthermore, I knew my burden was just beginning. The full impact of the news had not yet hit him. I knew what the future held and I had to guide him into it. A myriad of questions loomed. Shall I discuss them now or wait until they are raised?

He will probably ask, "Will I be cured? What will the treatments be like? What are the side effects, how long will they last? How much time will be lost from work? How much will treatment cost?" These questions imply hope and a positive attitude. But sometimes the more realistic questions are avoided: "Will I die? When?" Many patients will not voice this fear and some who do fail to hear the answers. Others fall apart when told. It is up to us to know how to respond. We must know when the other hard questions must be addressed, when to bring them up, and when to let the patient raise them: "How long will I live productively? Will there be pain and suffering? How will this affect my family—my wife, children, friends? What expenses can I anticipate: doctors, nurses, drugs, hospitalization, tests, help at home, nursing homes? What will my insurance cover? What will happen to my savings?"

These are just some of the problems Bob and his family face. Yes, there are occasional dramatic responses to therapy, but the probability is that Bob will eventually die from his cancer and he will need a lot of help along the way. His surgeon must provide much of it. He must furnish the guidance and initial advice. He must provide a feeling of hope and confidence in the results of planned therapy. He must help select oncologists, but not delegate responsibility too soon. He must continue to schedule office visits. If the treatments seem ineffective, he will be asked about other opinions and treatments. He must counsel the patient away from unsubstantiated and fraudulent practices. In time, others, the oncologists or family physician, may take over much of the surgeon's role, but the patient should never feel abandoned by his surgeon. The man who operated has a responsibility long after the last sutures are tied. He must stick with his patient to the very end. He should be there to answer questions, consult with others, participate in therapeutic decisions, and see his patient as often as required.

Such an approach calls upon the practice of the art of medicine — which means sensitivity and kindness. Truth must not be withheld, but it can be delivered gently and with tact. The issues being faced are fundamental and can't be shirked, nor must they be bluntly dealt with face on. On occasion, there is a place for half-truths, white lies, and kind deception. What these are cannot be taught or spelled out, but must become part of the humanity of being a doctor. Although surgeons are essentially manual technicians, they are also ministers of health and practitioners of a noble art.

15

THE DISCLOSURE OF INCURABILITY AND THE NEED FOR INTERDISCIPLINARY CARE—WHO IS IN CHARGE?

DAVID V. HABIF

Today, most patients who learn that they have a malignancy are eager to undergo treatment for cure. On the other hand, many patients who are told that they have incurable cancer, will conclude at the outset, before they know all of the facts, that pain, suffering, economic loss and a fatal outcome will be their fate within a short period of time. Very often the family will become involved in any decision making, once again before all of the necessary information about the disease has been given. In addition, both the patient and the family are influenced by friends and relatives who profess to know all there is to know about the disease and to offer advice freely. The lay press, radio, and television continue to give the public a great deal of information about cancer, including statistics concerning survival, and so forth. Finally, patients, families, insurance companies, and unions who pay medical insurance benefits are demanding and now are requiring second opinions for elective surgery.

Let us consider briefly the personality of patients who have incurable cancer, and how it tends to influence management. There are two broad groups of patients: the first is made up of those who wish to be in charge of their care, and the second is composed of those who wish to have guidance and decisions made for them. Patients in the first group are usually self-confident, decisive, independent, and do not wish to delegate authority for decision making to a physician or physicians. They wish to maintain control and, while they may respect physicians, they do not trust them completely. They will often seek multiple opinions, frequently within one specialty. Such patients will do well when the disease is not too severe, the treatment is not too intensive, or death is not expected in the near future. However, when one or more of these situations develops, many of these patients wish that a physician were in charge or would take charge.

The second group of patients wants a physician in charge to provide guidance, direction, and comfortable long-term survival. They are able to do this because their primary goal is getting better, rather than control, and they respect and trust their physician. They often do not wish to know all about the disease and to have discussions that belabor the information about a fatal outcome. They are grateful for the under-standing and the care which they receive.

Which physicians will take care of our patients? The Primary Physi-cian should be a Family Practitioner, an Internist, a Medical Oncologist, a Pediatric Oncologist, a Neurologist, and, in some cases, a Surgical Oncologist. The Primary Physician must assume the responsibility for the care of the patient over-all and should select all Consultants. They, in turn, should work through him and report to him and he must become the Captain of the team. The Primary Physician must have broad knowledge of the disease, he must understand the patient's person-ality and devote the necessary time to his care. He needs fine judgment and wisdom to perform this task and, additionally, he must have a strong personality. He may have to change consultants who will not work through him, and he must insist on unified care rather than fragmented treatment of the disease. He is in charge.

How often do we see this ideal treatment plan? Unfortunately, not very often and there are a variety of reasons. (1) The Primary Physician may not want to be the Captain and assume the responsibility. (2) The patient may not wish to incur the added expense, and (3) Consultants may wish to deal directly with the patient only. Frequently, Medical Oncologists will assume responsibility not only for treatment of the disease, but also for the patient as a whole. However, even they will not become involved in total patient care when a good deal of general medical care is required. The same is true of the Surgeon Oncologist, the Pediatric Oncologist, and the Neurologist.

It is my thesis that the patient with incurable cancer is best taken care of by a Primary Physician who is in charge and who takes charge. He will direct the patient, the consultants, and all of the allied health personnel involved. Anything short of this is a compromise.

16

THE NEED FOR NONSURGICAL CARE— SHIFTING RESPONSIBILITIES

Robert DeBellis

With the advent of alternative methods of therapy as care appropriate for the treatment of cancer patients, including in particular chemotherapy, the medical oncologist has assumed a larger role in the management of many post-surgical cancer patients. When called upon, the medical oncologist becomes involved, variously, at three different time periods—during the preoperative period, during the immediate postoperative period and, finally, during the long-term postoperative period when, in essence, he inherits the patient.

Regardless of when I start to deal with a patient, I regard it to be of utmost importance to find out from the patient exactly what he knows, what he has been told, what he is looking for in life, where he perceives he will be going, and what he knows about the extent of the disease. With this information, I can compassionately but realistically let patients know what I have to offer them and, above all, support a degree of optimism that allows a patient to function at whatever level he desires.

For several reasons an oncologist may see a patient during the preoperative period. As is becoming more and more evident in the lay press, everyone has become an authority on alternative care procedures in the treatment of malignancies—especially, for example, in the treatment of breast malignancies. The patient has many options—mastectomy, lumpectomy, radiotherapy, chemotherapy, combinations of these—if she chooses to be guided by the press. Perhaps she assures the surgeon that she knows what the diagnosis is. A modified radical mastectomy or a simple mastectomy with a node dissection has been proposed by her surgeon. The patient wants to know what the other alternatives are. She has concern about the surgeon: Can the surgeon be impartial? Isn't his interest only in surgery? Obviously, getting a second opinion from a nonsurgical person may be of benefit. Although, basically, I agree with the surgical approach to treatment of carcinoma of the breast, an open discussion of all the available options with their risks and benefits can be extremely beneficial for the patient. To hear from a nonsurgical professional that the surgical course of action is the best course of action is extremely helpful.

Another group of patients seeks medical oncologic consultation knowing that chemotherapy will follow surgery. They are anxious to pursue what might be involved or, perhaps, to become familiar with the doctor who is going to be treating them in the postoperative period. Today, everyone comes preprogrammed with concepts of chemotherapy. Our press does not do it justice. Television cannot sell shows with patients in complete remission, without nausea, vomiting, or hair loss. Frequently, a great deal of reinterpretation must be done for the patient and explanations given of what really will happen, that a normal life can be resumed.

Some patients consult with me after having developed a second malignancy. Decisions have to be made. Should surgical intervention be carried out in view of a preexisting malignancy that might still be present, although in a state of remission? Is the second malignancy an extension of the earlier one or is it a new malignancy? For some patients with recurrent disease, a diagnosis must be established by some open biopsy technique or a complication must be attended to. For example, if a patient develops a pathologic fracture while on chemotherapy, a decision must be made about the opportune time to initiate orthopedic surgery or—if the surgery has already been performed—when should chemotherapy be resumed? What is necessary for the management of the patient and the problems that arise in the setting of recurrent pathologic disease?

Chemotherapy has rendered many inoperable tumors operable. We believe that chemotherapy can change a stage C carcinoma of the breast to stage B or A. When this occurs, the patient returns to the surgeon for what should be a successful operation. There is growing evidence also that chemotherapy preoperatively may make a difference between success or failure for the patient with a primary soft tissue sarcoma or osteogenic sarcoma. Usually, I have the responsibility of the initial treatment for these patients before they are turned over to the surgeon. Following the surgical period, the patient is transferred back to my care.

In those situations where no established form of chemotherapy has been shown to be of benefit, careful investigation is called for. Although the outlook may be dismal, preoperatively, by incorporating into the care regimen what we think is the best chemotherapy available we can evaluate two different parameters. First, we are able to see if the chemotherapy has had any killing effect on the tumor which will be resected. Second, if it has been effective, a case can be made for continuing chemotherapy during the postoperative period. Our hope is to convert the patient who might not be cured by surgery into one who potentially might be cured by surgery.

When I have had opportunities to see patients preoperatively, a good introduction has been made to my involvement with them postoperatively. In the immediate postoperative period, I become a visitor and drop by to see the patient on a daily basis. I become a known quantity, another caring professional who, at that time and in some undefined way, is meaningfully keeping track of how things are going. The patient becomes a known quantity for me as well and my review of the chart sometimes reveals fine points that can be modified to help the patient through a particularly difficult period. Obviously, during this period the surgeon remains in charge, the captain of the ship, with the other medical personnel available to assist, perhaps to help make such decisions as whether radiotherapy should be introduced, when and if chemotherapy should be introduced. The surgeon is involved in the day-to-day management of the patient. His goal is to get the patient well enough to go home. He is fully cognizant that chemotherapy may be advisable postoperatively. When the chemotherapy has been similarly involved, it becomes possible to initiate chemotherapy in close proximity to the day the patient is scheduled to be discharged. Hospital bed utilization, efficiency, costs, and so forth can be positively affected by collaborative planning regarding initiation of chemotherapy postoperatively.

I feel that I play the greatest role when the patient has been smoothly shifted from surgical care to oncologic care—and this, we hope, will be a very long-term association. At this time, the patient is no longer primarily a surgical patient but has become the responsibility of another principal member of the caregiving team.

17

PSYCHIATRIC CONSULTATION
WITH THE INCURABLY ILL

MAHLON S. HALE, CONSTANCE WEISKOPF, AND ELIZABETH RAND

From my (M.S.H.) psychiatric residency in the early 1970s until this present time, my thinking about the role of the psychiatric consultant in working with dying patients has undergone numerous changes. These changes have been partly philosophical. As I grow older, I find myself becoming more stoical about death, particularly in a hospital that receives many referrals for protocols and treatment of the chronically ill. These changes are also partly the consequence of practice and experience with the problems other, more primary physicians, face with the dying and particularly with those patients vigorously treated who then turn incurable. And as I say this, I recognize the anomaly in using the word "turn" as though there were something wrong and inappropriate that any patient should do this. Thus, while our consultation team now performs more consultations around issues of death and dying than we did when our service evolved, our efforts have become refined in a practical sense, particularly when it comes to "doing things" and "setting goals." This is, in fact, because "incurability" seems to loom as a larger issue throughout the entire health care system to which we consult. At first I rationalized that these changes resulted from our coping mechanisms alone and had little to do with the behavior of the physicians and staffs with whom we consulted. Working with dying patients, even from a position that some physicians with primary responsibilities might justifiably view as tangential and protected, was stressful. This was so whether one was the attending, the service's nurse clinician, or a resident tran-

103

sient to our service. Perhaps psychiatrists and their mental health associates were different as those interminable jokes say. But I now think that this is not so, and infer that our behavior and resultant positioning of our consultation service must have other causes. Perhaps the fact that the philosophical bedrock of our specialty is uncertainty is the major contributing factor. When you are in a profession where the outcomes of interventions are often unclear and not predictable, you quickly learn not to expect certainty, even though one's views may be expressed in a manner that conveys assuredness.

From an experiential perspective, this refocusing is also the consequence, I believe, of our observing degrees of frustration and eventually uncertainty from referring physicians, services, patients, and their families that exceed what we are normally accustomed to see in those systems. And perhaps this requires some brief explanation. While it may be axiomatic to those physicians who resort to psychiatric consultants that identification of some psychological aspect to a patient's illness is a *prima facie* reason for calling a psychiatric consult, a different axiom operates for us. Very consistently, we find our services requested when some uncertainty has arisen in a physician's mind regarding some aspect of a patient. There are, of course, multiple possibilities. The doctor may not like the patient; or the patient may dislike the doctor. A patient may not get along with a roommate or the nursing staff. Peripheral complaints may exceed what is normally expected in such cases. Requests for tranquilizers, hypnotics, or analgesics are also routine reasons, as is the suspicion of manifest psychopathology. And occasionally a patient does ask to talk with a psychiatrist. But hidden among these routine reasons is the phenomenon of "not getting better," and just behind is "getting worse."

These conclusions may be made by anyone involved in the system; sometimes they are even made by us sitting on the sidelines, wondering whether we will be called in. Perhaps it is a healthy adjustment to personal experiences, both good and bad, and to the realities of "unhealth" and disease, to be able to say that a patient is not getting better, or even getting worse. But few of us like to acknowledge it, and none of us would wish it on ourselves. When such observations come to represent the beliefs of our consultees, a substantial task is imposed on the psychiatrist, particularly as these beliefs are not, or cannot, always be verbalized. Let me hasten to add that I do not want to suggest that our consultees are remiss in raising the issues surrounding incurable illness. But their stake, if you will, like the stake of their patients is different from ours, and I cannot help but think that this wears terribly at them and raises the spectre that raising the issue of incurability is tantamount to "giving up." The case we now present illustrates many of these points.

Several months ago we were asked to see a forty-year-old woman with a three-month history of thrombocytopenia and new onset leukopenia. The patient was a housewife and mother from a surrounding community who had never been significantly ill medically or psychiatrically. The consult request, which emphasized that she was intractable to "all conventional treatments for ITP," was initiated by her hematologist, who found her depressed and difficult to manage. We found the patient indeed depressed. She was very angry and demanding as well. She quickly expressed her upset regarding her treatment, diagnosis, and day-to-day management. It soon became clear that she was understandably frightened by the failure of all treatments to date to arrest her downhill course and its multiple complications. Her own uncertainty was revealed when she reported, "I don't think I'll die of the illness, but I may die of the complications."

Although she was Cushingoid, we felt that her mood followed logically from her condition as well as her lengthy separation from her young children and husband, and her coping style followed from her preexisting personality. We elected to intervene both in consultant and liaison capacities, that is in dialogue with the patient as well as with the ongoing system of care. With the caregivers at this stage, we adopted the conventional maneuver of suggesting that one member of the team become the intermediary or spokesman for medical information, a maneuver that at once becomes more essential and more problematic as the number of caregivers increases, as it will where there is uncertainty. In fact, the patient said to us that she could "hear uncertainty in the voices of [my] doctors." Our goal was to avoid the multiple, changing communications the patient had been receiving and to assure her a constant contact. Her subsequent choices for spokesmen reflected their own ready access to the emotional impact of the patient's predicament.

In the course of our dialogue with the patient as the first, now "experimental treatment" failed, and the holidays came and went leaving her more ill than ever, she passed through an amalgam of phases of dying. These we addressed with her, in the course of which she abruptly sent indirect word that she wished no further contact with us. After we explored this response with her, however, she "rewelcomed" us. At this point, our liaison function focused on addressing the frustration and uncertainty of the medical staff, encouraging and enabling them to be more upfront with the patient. Her vivid quotation, "I feel like each part of my body is dying slowly," came to summarize accurately her feeling state and eventually the feelings of the physicians caring for her. We tried to use this awareness and perspective to redefine for the staff the patient's psychological state as one of dying. It became clear that the patient was telling us where "she was at," we were listening and translating, and all the caregivers were running to catch up with the patient psychologically.

Eventually, this patient was transfered to a medical center in New York for a research protocol unavailable with us. At the time of her transfer, she was substantially worse, but hopeful as were her primary physicians who looked for "a successful treatment." As she left, our staff was able to voice their relief at now sharing the burden of this extremely distressing case. Several weeks later, the patient was transferred back to our hospital with the report that she had responded well and would only require maintenance of her regimen followed by her discharge home. But as with all previous interventions, this initial favorable response was rapidly followed by relapse to a more serious condition. Psychiatry was called in again, not at a time correlated with a change in the patient's mood, but rather at the moment this new treatment was seen to fail. In fact, on readmission the patient had changed. She was no longer a management problem in terms of anger or demands. In response to our observation regarding these changes, she told us "I don't have so many feelings any more." In spite of our efforts to enable her to talk about dying with us and her husband, she was reluctant, in part she said because she had not been given a terminal diagnosis. The problem in acknowledging incurability affected her management to the very end. When she became obtunded and intubated in the ICU, our role remained both that of liaison and consultation psychiatrists. Having assessed the family's readiness to accept a negative outcome at this point, we turned to the question of sustaining her life with the medical house staff. In spite of a clear statement that there were no further experimental regimens to offer this patient, there remained a reluctance to acknowledge that the patient was incurable "because of her age and the absence of a final diagnosis." Thus, it was only minutes before her death that the decision was made not to attempt resuscitation.

Consultation-liaison work around issues of dying and more specifically around incurability inevitably requires shifting of gears and expectations on the part of requesting physicians, staffs, patients, families, and psychiatrists. This is an uncomfortable experience for all involved. Psychiatrists are aware as well that they are sometimes called when other remedies have failed, and that referring physicians may have lowered their expectations vis à vis results or cure. They are also aware of the many pressures, even social pressures, that bear upon decisions to continue treatments in incurable cases. It is unfortunate that there continues to be some reluctance to call upon us in such cases as I have described. As the clouds of incurability gather, other consultants are often called for in such numbers that sometimes one loses track as to who literally is in charge of the primary care of the patient. Inevitably this is one way of losing focus.

While psychiatry as a discipline has no special skills in facilitating the linear process that envelops much of medicine, psychiatrists do have certain skills in making global assessments, in determining where an individual or a system is focused, and where it is diffuse. In a way, we might conceptualize psychiatric consultants as being relatively unencumbered by the linearity of decision making and caregiving that others specialize in. Put another way, we do have some skills in getting others to step back and take a look at the whole problem. In spite of our consultation, results can be variable and sometimes undesired. Our presence, however, can aid others in refocusing their caregiving particularly where the issue of incurability has become manifest.

18

RADIATION THERAPY IN THE CONTINUING CARE OF THE INCURABLE PATIENT

JEAN M. BARSA

X-rays were discovered in 1895 by Konrad Roentgen. Immediately thereafter it was applied not only in the diagnosis of diseases, but also in the treatment of malignant diseases. As a new tool in the hand of the medical profession, it was used in the treatment of a variety of diseases including arthritis and different skin conditions. The technological advances were rapidly progressing, but the biological knowledge was slowly accumulating pointing not only to the beneficial effect of x-rays, but also to its side effects. E.H. Grubbe claimed to have treated a patient with cancer of the breast in January of 1896. In the same year, Voigt in Germany treated a patient with cancer for the relief of pain; luckily he was out of the reach of the FDA. In 1896, the Curies discovered radium and it was used in 1903 for the first time in containers in the uterus and in 1905 as an interstitial implant in the treatment of malignant diseases.

Clinically, radiation therapy was born in 1922 when Regaud, Coutard, and others started to use the 200 KV x-rays tubes in the treatment of patients with cancer. Cancer of the larynx was one of the first successfully treated cancers. In the 1930s high energy machines were developed. In the 1950s the Cobalt 60 machine was introduced and in the 1960s the linear accelerators. The advantage of all of these machines is that they can deliver a radiation dose to the deep structure of the body with skin-sparing effect, that is with little damage to the overlying skin.

One has to look at the cancer statistics in order to appreciate the role of radiation therapy in the management of patients with cancer, whether it is a primary, adjunctive, or palliative modality. The overall incidence of cancer in the United States, excluding skin and in situ cancer, is about 340 cases per 100,000 population. The death rate is about 170 per 100,000 population. Of these patients with cancer, approximately two-thirds will require radiation therapy at one point or another during their life. In the majority of cases the treatment is of palliative value mainly for the relief of pain.

Briefly, I would like to present a short summary of the nature and effect of ionizing radiation.

The ionizing radiation is either electromagnetic in nature like x-rays and gamma rays or corpuscular like electrons, protons, and alpha particles. The ionizing radiation is either natural like the gamma rays emanating from radium or artificial like the one produced by the x-ray and Cobalt 60 machines.

The effect of ionizing radiation on living matter can be divided into two components. The first is the physical-chemical reaction secondary to deposition of energy in the absorbing material; the second is the biological effect which is much longer in duration and forms the basis for radiation therapy. It takes advantage of the radio-vulnerability of tumor cells in comparison to normal cells and the ability of the normal cells to recover from radiation injuries.

Radiation therapy plays a major role in the treatment of cancer whether it is alone as in the treatment of cancer of the larynx or cervix or as an adjunctive modality in the treatment of head and neck cancer and cancer of the uterus. Radiation therapy is also the single most effective palliative treatment in the symptomatic dying patient. Pain is the major symptom in the dying patient caused either by the growing tumor or by metastases, whether it is metastases to bones, lungs, brain, or other organs. Unfortunately, sometimes a patient is referred to the radiation therapy department only after analgesics have become ineffective in controlling pain. The response rate to palliative radiation therapy for the relief of pain varies with the underlying disease. For metastatic carcinoma of the kidney it is about 30–50 percent. In metastatic carcinoma of the lung, prostate, and colon it is about 50–80 percent. The response rate in pain from metastatic carcinoma from the breast is well over 90 percent. It is a gratifying experience to see a patient suffering agonizing pain from metastatic breast cancer to the spine becoming, after a few treatments, asymptomatic and able to ambulate and care for herself. It is indeed remarkable how sometimes after a few treatments to a cord compression from metastatic disease, a patient could regain control over the functions of his legs. Hemoptysis in a patient with advanced cancer of the lung can be stopped with radiation therapy. In 1970 a dying patient with advanced cancer of the lung measuring about 15 cm. in diameter was brought to our department coughing literally cups of blood. He was begging for help so that he could live a little bit longer. After two weeks of treatment not only did the bleeding stop, but he lived three more years of productive life and died of a heart attack.

As physicians, it is our duty if we cannot cure a patient with cancer because of its advanced stage, to at least render his remaining time as pain-free and comfortable as possible. The majority of patients are not afraid of dying. What they fear is suffering. It is the quality of life, rather than its duration that should be the prime concern of the medical profession. Dying is the only certainty in life and dying in patients with cancer is a little bit more certain. Radiation therapy is a major contributor to the easing of the transition between life and death in the patient with incurable cancer.

A patient dying of incurable cancer finds himself, when brought into a hospital, in a strange environment, full of large and small machines and among strangers. His psychological loneliness is overwhelming and he needs human compassion in addition to whatever bodily relief we can offer.

19

ETHICAL ISSUES IN SURGICAL INTERVENTION: SOCIAL WORKER AS ADVOCATE

ELIZABETH J. CLARK

Oncology social work as a specialty is not a new concept. In 1937 Eleanor Cockerill, a pioneer in social work with cancer patients, published an article entitled "The Social Worker Looks at Cancer." She discussed the problems that cancer patients face and grouped them into three main areas:

1. There is the concrete, objective need for adequate medical care — which may or may not be available depending upon the resources of the patient and his community;
2. There are those problems relating to environmental adjustments which become necessary because of the patient's illness; and
3. There are the deeper emotional problems that arise out of the patient's struggle to cope with the disease.

A decade later (1948–50), a research project that considered "The Emotional Problems of Patients with Cancer" was conducted at Massachusetts General Hospital. This led to Ruth Abrams' article on "Social Case Work with Cancer Patients" (1951) in which she described the role of the case worker in oncology:

> The case worker, as a member of the professional group, has by the very nature of his function and training, the best opportunity to study and to contribute to the evaluation of the attitudes of the patient with cancer and to give him sustained and planned support where and when this is indicated (p. 434).

The works and writings of both Eleanor Cockerill and Ruth Abrams emphasize the role of the social worker in oncology, and implicit in their work is the concept of advocacy. Yet, 30 to 40 years after the pioneering work of these women, there seems to be less emphasis placed on the concept of advocacy in oncology and in other social work areas. In fact, in this age of specialization, with so many professionals involved at so many levels, some hospitals have found it necessary to create a special position called "patient advocate" or "patients' right advocate" whose primary responsibility is advising patients about their health care rights and how to assert and protect them (Barry 1982). What used to be an integral part of social casework skills has become another area of specialization.

Social work itself has become more and more specialized. There are currently such differentiations as clinical social workers, psychiatric social workers, and oncology social workers, to name only a few. The generic term of "case worker" has lost favor as the functions of the social worker have become more specialized, narrower, and somewhat restricted.

This is not to imply that oncology social workers do not need specialized knowledge. They do (Blum and Euster-Fisher, 1983). Just as one would expect a certain specialized knowledge base and expertise from social workers on a cardiac unit or a neurosurgery unit, the same would be expected of social workers who work primarily on an oncology unit or with cancer patients. They need to know as much as possible about cancer as a disease, treatments used, possible side effects, and the social and psychological problems that frequently accompany the illness. But becoming knowledgeable about these topics should not overshadow the importance of the basic tenets of social work practice—client self-determination and advocacy.

ADVOCACY

Advocacy, in the classical sense means "summoning to one's assistance, defending, or calling to one's aid" (Barry 1982:187). A useful definition for advocacy in health care is "the act of informing and supporting persons, so that they can make the best decisions possible for themselves" (Kohnke 1980:2038).

It is the role and responsibility of social work advocacy in surgical oncology that this paper will address. However, to talk about advocacy, it is first necessary to mention the rights of patients and the responsibilities of social workers that these rights imply.

Wellman defines a "right" as "a claim or sphere of decision that is, or ought to be, respected by other individuals and protected by society. A responsibility is a sphere of duty or obligation assigned to a person by the nature of that person's position, function, or work (Wellman 1975:252).

Within a patient's rights framework, eleven rights of surgical oncology patients, which also imply social work responsibility, can be discussed.

Right #1: The Right to Know the Diagnosis and Prognosis.

The philosophy of telling cancer patients their diagnosis has reversed itself in the last decade. In the 1960s, there was a strong tendency not to tell patients they had cancer (Oken 1961), but recent compelling evidence (McIntosh 1974; Novak et al. 1979) indicates that patients wish to be told the truth regarding their illnesses. This trend of disclosure appears to coincide with the patients' rights movement and with the tightening of regulations of informed consent procedures for malpractice purposes.

In 1973, the American Hospital Association released "A Patient's Bill of Rights" which most hospitals in the United States have subsequently adopted in some form. One right concerns disclosure of the patient's diagnosis:

> The patient has the right to obtain from his physician complete current information concerning his diagnosis, treatment, and prognosis in terms the patient can be reasonably expected to understand.

Agreeing that patients have a right to know their diagnosis, and as far as possible their prognosis, does not mean that there is a consensus about specific guidelines for the telling nor the timing of such information. It is generally understood that each situation needs to be evaluated, and hope appropriate to the circumstances extended. But who should do the telling, who should be present, the amount of detail included, and the language used is less easily determined. Cancer patients are often overwhelmed with the initial diagnosis of cancer, and may not be able to grasp any additional information. Therefore, explaining treatment plans in detail at the time of the initial telling is often futile and will need to be repeated later, perhaps several times, before they can be understood.

In providing support for the patient, having a social worker present at the time of relaying the diagnosis can be very useful. Additionally, the time of diagnosis is a crucial intervention point for social work practice with oncology patients. The social worker can remain with the patient and family when the physician leaves, and she can begin to assess their coping style and abilities, and can also evaluate not only what they have understood about the information the physician provided, but also what other areas need further emphasis.

Clarification is important at the time of diagnosis. The average patient and family have many misconceptions about cancer. They generally equate cancer with death and see a cancer diagnosis as a death sentence. This is due mainly to what Sontag calls "the stigma of cancer." She stresses that both society and health care professionals contribute to this stigma, and notes (1978: 7–8):

As long as a particular disease is treated as an evil, invincible predator, not just a disease, most people with cancer will indeed be demoralized by learning what disease they have. The solution is hardly to stop telling patients the truth, but to rectify the conception of the disease, to demythicize it.

Social workers trained in oncology are especially adept at helping patients and their family members put cancer as a disease into perspective. The sooner this is done, the better able the patient is to move forward with the treatment process, and the more supportive and hopeful the family can be in this process.

Right #2. The Right to be Fully Informed of the Benefits and Risks of a Surgical Procedure in Terms Which the Patient Can Understand.

Right #3. The Right to Acquire a Second Opinion, Including That of the Pathologist, Prior to Surgery.

Right #4. The Right to Information About Alternative Treatments and the Right to Time for Deliberation.

Rights #2, 3, and 4 are based on the principle of self-determination, a fundamental value to which social workers have historically had a strong commitment. The Code of Ethics of the National Association of Social Workers (1980) states that "the social worker should make every effort to foster maximum self-determination on the part of clients."

Nowhere is the oncology social worker's role as advocate more important than in the area of information transmission regarding the issues of informed consent and alternative treatments.

There has been much debate about the nature and limitations of informed consent. Two factors are usually noted as being essential if consent is to be truly informed. The first is deliberation, and the second is free choice. This means that patients must understand what they are consenting to and must then voluntarily choose it (Barry 1982). In order to do this, they need not only enough information, but information that is comprehensible and usable. Often patients are provided information which is so technical that instead of understanding it, they are intimidated by it. Also, as Annas (1975) has noted, the physician can phrase scientific information in such a way as to predetermine the patient's decision. Additionally, informed consent forms are generally designed for the legal protection of the hospital and health care professional, not for readability on the patient's part.

Frequently, a physician or a health care professional will go over an informed consent form in some detail with the patient. At the conclusion, the patient is asked if there are any questions; often none are asked. This is not proof that they understood what was said, but may well indicate that they did not understand enough or are too frightened of the procedure to ask questions. An important function of the social worker in informed consent is helping the patient and the family to formulate the questions that they want to ask. This means helping them interpret the information and putting it in a form that is usable from the patient's perspective.

Additionally, in health care settings, there is a habit of prejudging a patient's capacity to understand information. This occurs despite the fact that most hospital records relate little about a patient's educational background, and few physicians or health care professionals explore this area. The social worker is the member of the health care team best trained to assess the educational and emotional resources that the patient and family possess and, through frequent contact, can evaluate the patient's level of understanding and need for periodic and additional information.

The amount and form of information needed will vary with the educational level and familiarity with medical terms and procedures of each patient, and there is agreement that the information must be individualized. In this way, more care is being taken to see that consent is more informed. However, there is still much debate regarding the patient's capability to choose between alternative methods of treatment.

The argument against providing the patient with information with regard to alternative treatments is still based on the fact that medicine is highly scientific, esoteric and requires an extremely technical vocabulary (Alfidi 1971). As a result, the argument continues, patients are not capable of making their own informed choices, and are better off if the physician decides.

In the past, this argument has been used extensively when determining treatment for breast cancer. As a result, alternative treatments were not mentioned to the patients. Several states no longer allow this paternalistic attitude with regard to breast cancer treatment. Five states (California, Hawaii, Wisconsin, Massachusetts, and Minnesota) require physicians to inform their patients of all alternative effective methods before proceeding with treatment. California requires that the women be given a seven page written summary so that they can make an intelligent and informed consent. The California brochure also includes a statement that it is appropriate to seek an additional opinion prior to surgery, and that "it is very important to take a reasonable amount of time to obtain enough medical information and consultation to make a final and informed decision" (Roberti 1983:3).

Providing patients with adequate information about surgical procedures and possible alternative treatments will not ensure that they choose the treatment that the physician feels is the best, but it generally will ensure that patients will choose the treatment or procedure that they feel is best for them.

Not infrequently, the social worker is placed in the role of "persuader," and is assigned the task of convincing an objecting patient to sign a consent form for a specific treatment or to help the patient realize the value of the treatment procedure which the physician sees as optimal. A social worker can be very effective in this role because she usually understands the patient's limitations and vulnerabilities. However, "siding with" the physician, and using her skills to manipulate the patient to arrive at a pre-determined decision runs counter to the social work principle of client self-determination.

When a patient refuses a certain procedure, or any treatment at all, the stakes are even higher and the role of the social worker becomes complex.

Right #5. The Right to Refuse a Surgical Procedure, and the Right to Receive Adequate Counseling and Support During and After the Decision-Making Period.

Ethicists have become concerned about the rightness of intervention. The past two decades have seen numerous ethical questions raised about such topics as euthanasia, abortion, living wills, and brain-death legislation. Many of these issues are a direct result of the patients' rights movement. Advocacy involves making certain patients are aware of their rights, and these rights include refusal of treatment.

What is the role of the social worker when a patient refuses a treatment, or refuses all treatment? Foremost, she must see to it that the patient has all relevant facts and information necessary to make the decision. This will, of course, entail arranging for the patient and family to speak with persons who can help place the decision in perspective and can provide the needed information. The act of informing is the first part of advocacy. The second part is supporting the patient once the decision has been reached. This includes not only reassuring patients that it is their decision and that they have the right to make it, but also that they will be supported regardless of the unpopularity of their choice or the pressures exerted by hospital, physician, family, friends, or other health care professionals.

Supporting may involve actions or nonactions, and Kohnke (1980) suggests that nonactions may be even more important than actions, and harder to accomplish (Barry 1982:188):

Nonaction usually means keeping oneself from subtly undercutting the patient's decisions. It may also involve refusing the requests of others . . . to talk to patients and convince them they are wrong.

Being an advocate in this situation is especially difficult when one's training and knowledge do not agree with the patient's decision. Equally difficult is going against the physician's or the hospital's recommendations. The major functions of advocacy can frequently be at odds with the culture of the hospital system (Barry 1982), but that does not change the social worker's responsibility to the patient and his or her right to self-determination.

Right #6. The Right to Pre-Operative Counseling and Support Once a Decision to Undergo the Surgical Procedure Has Been Made.

Right #7. The Right to Expect Support for Family Members Before, During and After the Surgical Procedure.

Right #8. The Right to Optimal PostOperative Care Including Information, Instruction and Pain Control.

Most patients are apprehensive about any surgical intervention, but for cancer patients, the preoperative period is characterized by anxiety and depression greater than is usual for patients anticipating general types of major surgery (Hardy and Cull 1975). The patient may be uncooperative and demanding, and reassurances may frequently fall on deaf ears. Therefore, it cannot be stated too strongly that preoperative counseling is of inestimable value.

This counseling should include the patient's spouse and immediate family who are themselves unsure of the situation and often uninformed about what to expect postoperatively. This uncertainty of those around the patient only contributes to his or her apprehension and anxiety.

Some preoperative fear is normal and even desirable as it may help the patient and family understand and plan for what the postoperative period will entail. Janis (1958) found that very unanxious preoperative patients were at higher risk for postoperative problems than persons who were somewhat apprehensive, and that they were frequently masking their fears. Other studies (Egbert and Battit 1964; Smith 1976) found that preoperative counseling helps to reduce certain surgical complications and may reduce the amount of postoperative medication required and the length of the postoperative hospital stay.

Social workers can ascertain the patient's and family's fears and misconceptions about the surgery. Some of these the social worker can allay, while others will need to be referred to the surgeon who will perform the procedure. For patients who are especially anxious, the surgeon's preoperative discussion should take place in several visits, thus giving the patient and family time to absorb the information and to formulate questions. Discussion should include expected postoperative pain and discomfort, bodily changes that will occur, how long the patient will be in the hospital, the outlook for recovery, and possible problems with future functioning at both physical and social levels.

The family should be supported during the surgical procedure. Often they are at a loss about their role during this time. It is easy to tell them to go home, and that a staff member or the surgeon will call when the operation is over. Most families, however, wish to remain at the hospital. For many, this tends to alleviate some of their anxiety because they feel closer to their loved one and on-hand if an emergency should arise. Special consideration should be given to these family members, including a designated waiting area, and frequent contacts with the social worker who was part of the preoperative counseling team will give them a feeling of continuity and help them to keep their anxiety at a manageable level.

When the surgery is completed, privacy should be provided for the surgeon to report the outcome to the family members, especially so if the news is not favorable. Here again, the social worker's presence can be an asset. She can remain with the family to be supportive and help them to adjust to the news and the situation.

Once the surgery is over, the process of coping with the injury to the body begins. Pain, obviously, needs to be controlled, and both the patient and the family need to know what is normal and what is expected of them during the immediate postoperative period. Additionally, the patient and family will require help in dealing with their emotional response to the illness and the surgery, particularly if there has been an amputation or a loss of function which will preclude a return to a preoperative level of physical or social activity.

The health care team and the social worker can assist the patient and the family in the adaptive and rehabilitative stages by continuing the emotional support and education that began preoperatively.

The social worker plays a particularly important role in the discharge planning process. She assesses the patient's family situation and their ability to care for the patient at home, and arranges assistance where necessary. Particular attention must be given to patients who are reluctant to leave the hospital and to families who are reluctant to have the patient return home. Oftentimes, the patient has come to feel dependent on the hospital staff, particularly the nurses, and the family may doubt their ability to provide optimal care at home. These fears can usually be reduced by education, support, and by the knowledge that the family can contact the physician or social worker if a question or emergency arises.

Right #9. The Right to Adequate Prosthetic Devices.

Right #10. The Right to Information About Reconstructive Surgery
Regardless of Age or Stage of Disease.

If an amputation has occurred or if the disease or the surgical proce-dure has resulted in a need for a prosthetic device, every effort should be made to obtain this for the patient. Frequently with cancer, financial concerns are prohibitive, and good prosthetic devices are expensive. For example, for a female breast cancer patient over the age of 65, the only means of acquiring a breast prosthesis may be her Medicare reimburse-ment. Past experience has indicated that Medicare reimburses about half the cost of a good, wellfitted breast prosthesis. Helping a patient acquire an optimal prosthesis will require resourcefulness, creativity, and deter-mination on the part of the social worker.

The same type of advocacy may be necessary to help obtain reconstruc-tive surgery for a patient, and education for staff can help. Not long ago, a surgical oncologist and a plastic surgeon were giving a talk at a cancer patient support meeting to a group of women who had undergone mastectomies. They used slides which showed how effective breast recon-struction could be after a mastectomy. The support group was composed primarily of women over age 50, many of whom had been patients of the surgical oncologist. None of the women over age 50 had had reconstruc-tive surgery, nor even had it discussed with them, but several younger women in the group had had it, or had spoken with the plastic surgeon about it. When the physicians were questioned about this difference, it became apparent that they thought only women under age 45 would be interested, and, therefore, it had not occurred to them to suggest it to older women. Since that time, several of the over-fifty women in that group have had breast reconstruction performed.

This is not to suggest that reconstructive surgery is an option for every cancer patient. However, cancer patients do have a right to obtain infor-mation about the possibility of such a procedure, and no arbitrary limits of age nor stage of disease should be set as the determining factors for discussing this service.

Another interesting discrepancy with regard to reconstructive surgery was that previously some medical insurance policies would not reim-burse for breast reconstruction for female cancer patients on the basis that it was strictly cosmetic surgery. However, testicular reconstruction for male cancer patients was a reimbursable expense. It took some advocacy skills to get this discriminatory practice discontinued, and both procedures are now reimbursable.

Right #11. The Right to Rehabilitative Services to the Fullest Extent Possible,
Regardless of Incurability of Disease.

A broad definition of the term "rehabilitation" in connection with cancer treatment is given by Holland and Frei (1973: 498):

> Rehabilitation is a continuing part of cancer management. It entails helping the patient adjust to an altered body image as well as limitations placed upon him by his disease and its treatment, *whether successful or not.* Proper management entails a commitment to achieving optimal patient function and satisfaction from life, during and after therapeutic procedures, *for as long as the patient lives.* (Emphasis added.)

Dietz (1969) refers to the concept of "palliative rehabilitation" when there is increasing disability from progressing disease.

Unfortunately, in the acute care environment of our modern hospital settings, availability of services and resources may often be limited. There is a tendency to provide care where it is felt it is most needed or where it will be most useful. With regard to rehabilitation programs, the incurable cancer patient may not fall in this category. These patients may require more assistance and advocacy on the part of the social worker to obtain rehabilitative services so that they can live as fully as possible, functioning as well as possible, despite the advanced stage of their illness.

SUMMARY

Eleven rights which address potential problem areas for cancer patients who need or undergo surgical intervention, and which demonstrate the importance of social work advocacy have been discussed. These include:

1. The right to know the diagnosis and prognosis.
2. The right to be fully informed of the benefits and risks of a surgical procedure in terms which the patient can understand.
3. The right to acquire a second opinion, including that of the pathologists, prior to surgery.
4. The right to information about alternative treatments and the right to time for deliberations.

5. The right to refuse a surgical procedure, and the right to receive adequate counseling and support during and after the decision-making period.
6. The right to preoperative counseling and support once a decision to undergo the surgical procedure has been made.
7. The right to expect support for family members before, during and after the surgical procedure.
8. The right to optimal postoperative care including information, instruction, and pain control.
9. The right to adequate prosthetic devices.
10. The right to information about reconstructive surgery regardless of age or stage of disease.
11. The right to rehabilitative services to the fullest extent possible, regardless of incurability of disease.

Advocacy, based on the premise of client self-determination, should be an important aspect of oncology social work. Yet, the specialization of social work today sometimes overshadows this function.

To be effective oncology social workers do need specialized knowledge and training about cancer and its concomitant problems. This expertise is necessary for informing and supporting cancer patients so they can make the best possible decisions for themselves.

There is a danger, however, that specialization leads to a restricted and narrow focus of intervention. In oncology social work this appears to result in an emphasis on the intrapsychic problems of cancer patients, with less attention being paid to the interpersonal or the community interactional, in other words the social problems that the patient experiences as a result of the illness, and the areas where advocacy is most needed.

Advocacy has been a cornerstone of social work practice, and is much too important to be delegated to another profession for the sake of specialization. Specialized knowledge should be a complement to basic social work practice skills. It should be an addition, not a replacement.

REFERENCES

Abrams, R. 1951. "Social Case Work with Cancer Patients." *Social Casework* 32: 425–435.
Alfidi, R. J. 1971. "Informed Consent: A Study of Patient Reaction." *Journal of the American Medical Association* 216: 1325–1329.

Annas, G. 1974. *The Rights of Hospital Patients.* New York: Avon Books.

Barry, V. 1982. *Moral Aspects of Health Care.* Belmont, CA: Wadsworth.

Blum, D. and S. Euster-Fisher. 1983. "Clinical Supervisory Practice in Oncology Settings." *The Clinical Supervisor* 1: 17–27.

Cockerill, E. 1937. "The Social Worker Looks at Cancer." *The Family.* New York: Family Service Association of America.

Dietz, J. H. 1969. "Rehabilitation of the Cancer Patient." *Medical Clinics of North America* 53: 3.

Egbert, L. and G. Battit. 1964. "Reduction of Postoperative Pain by Encouragement and Instruction of Patients: A Study of Doctor-Patient Rapport." *New England Journal of Medicine* 220: 825–827.

Hardy, R. and J. Cull. 1975. *Counseling and Rehabilitating the Cancer Patient.* Springfield: Charles C Thomas.

Holland, J. and E. Frei. 1973. *Cancer Medicine.* Philadelphia: Lea and Febiger.

Janis, I. 1958. *Psychological Stress: Psychoanalytic and Behavioral Studies of Surgical Patients.* New York: John Wiley and Sons, Inc.

Kohnke, M. F. 1980. "The Nurse as Advocate." *American Journal of Nursing* November: 2038.

McIntosh, J. 1974. "Process of Communication, Information Seeking and Control Associated with Cancer: A Selected Review of the Literature." *Social Science and Medicine* 8: 167–187.

National Association of Social Workers. 1980. Code of Ethics of the National Association of Social Workers. Washington, D.C: NASW.

Novak, D., R. Plummer, R. Smith, H. Ochtill, G. Morrow, and J. Bennett. 1979. "Changes in Physicians' Attitudes Toward Telling the Cancer Patient." *Journal of the American Medical Association* 241: 897–900.

Oken, D. 1961. "What to Tell Cancer Patients: A Study of Medical Attitudes." *Journal of the American Medical Association* 175: 1120–1128.

Roberti, D. 1983. *Breast Cancer Treatment: Summary of Alternative Effective Methods, Risks, Advantages and Disadvantages.* Sacramento: California Department of Health.

Smith, E. 1976. *A Comprehensive Approach to Rehabilitation of the Cancer Patient: A Self-Instructional Text.* New York: McGraw-Hill.

Sontag, S. 1978. *Illness as Metaphor.* New York: Vintage Books.

Wellman, C. 1975. *Morals and Ethics.* Glenview: Scott, Foresman.

20

WHO'S IN CHARGE: UNSHARED REALITIES

FLORENCE SELDER

INTRODUCTION

A proper response to the question of who is in charge regarding the disclosure of an incurable illness to a patient and the need for interdisciplinary care depends on what view of the world or perception of reality one adopts. In this chapter, at least two perceptions of reality and their corresponding characteristics will be described; the misunderstandings that occur from the interaction of these two perceptions and their implications for health professionals will be discussed.

PROCESS/NONPROCESS REALITIES

A perception of reality is the way a person relates to the world, i.e., institutions, systems, or other persons. The two perceptions of reality that are described here are process (infinite) and nonprocess (finite) realities.[1]

The framework that organizes a nonprocess perception of reality emanates from the person who is the center of that reality and simultaneously is the focus of the person's relationship to the world, i.e., the self and how the world relates to it. In some ways, a nonprocess perception is static as the position is located in a particular point in time.

In contrast, the process view of reality is organized by relationships, and these are central to the person's reality, i.e., the relationships and how these relate to the world. The latter position is dynamic as one is forever evolving in the interrelatedness of relating to the world and others.

The theme that organizes a nonprocess reality is that the most important aspect of one's reality is oneself or what one defines as oneself, i.e., one's work, one's children. Indeed, if one's self or one's work is of primary importance, then it follows that one views oneself as the one in charge either by virtue of who one is (e.g., physician) or by virtue of one's position in a system (e.g., chief of surgery). Frequently, the view of "being in charge" becomes nonnegotiable with members from any other discipline, with members within one's discipline, and certainly non-negotiable with the patient.

In contrast, the process view of reality is organized by the means that the person relates to the world, and this means is by the relationships that the person forms. The focus of relationships in a process reality is antithetical to the self as the center. From a process perception of reality, the question of who is in charge is answered simply by asking who can best facilitate whatever, whenever, wherever for whomever. Because the process perception is not static, the identified in-charge person will vary according to the needs of the patient in the health care system.

CHARACTERISTICS OF THE SYSTEMS

A characteristic of the nonprocess system is that it is hierarchal in organization. If the center of one's reality is oneself, then it is imperative to have a means by which one can locate oneself within a system. By locating where one fits within a system, one organizes that location in relation to others. In a nonprocess system, the location of oneself is usually in relationship to some ranking. Inherent in the ranking will be the designation of responsibilities, privileges, and status. In a hierarchical organization, there is a temptation to advocate one's responsibilities as the most important and to consider one's position in some lineage. In the process system, there is an absence of a hierarchal structure. The selection of the appropriate care provider in a patient-care situation will depend on the primacy of what the patient needs and who is skilled or, in the case of skill overlap, who is available to meet those needs.

Closely akin to a hierarchical system is the adherence to rules. Rules are a regulatory approach to others and support the institution/system. Rules may take precedence over the individual. Frequently, a person from a nonprocess perspective will want to run a hospital unit as a "tight-ship" with the self as captain. The interest in instituting rules and locating responsibility is that it is a means of reducing uncertainty and decreasing ambiguity. People operating from a process system cannot understand the reliance on rules. For example, the scheduling of surgery should be based on who is the one most in need and not by any protocol of surgeon ranking.

A second characteristic distinguishes the two perceptions, the assumption that underlies each reality. The assumption underlying the nonprocess perception of reality is that the reality must be perceived as dualistic. Simplifying the world as "either-or" is very efficient. If one is in charge, then others must not be in charge. However, once one chooses to be in charge, then no other alternative is conceptually feasible except what one does not choose, i.e., someone else to be in charge. Inherent in any dualistic system is a rightness or wrongness, a goodness or a badness, and a success or a failure. Health care providers develop elaborate rituals never to be wrong. The efforts made not to be wrong will comprise a variety of behaviors, i.e., distancing from the patient or transferring the patient to someone else's care.

A third characteristic that differentiates the two perceptions of reality is the way the individual considers information. An individual who adopts a nonprocess perspective would consider information in a linear progression until some conclusion is reached.[2] In the process system, the information is regarded in a multivariate or a multidimensional manner (this is sometimes termed horizontal thinking). Often, nonprocess thinking is described as logical and rational. Conversely, the process style is portrayed as scattered and irrelevant.[3]

In terms of the team concept in health care, another characteristic that contrasts the two realities is the concept of power. Power in the nonprocess system is seen as finite. Consequently, if power (i.e., space and territory, authority) is given to a hematologist, then one will have less power and will have to monitor that hematologist. Power in a process system is seen as infinite. Thus, if power is shared with other health professionals, then all persons will be more powerful.

UNDERSTANDING/MISUNDERSTANDING

The manner of caregiving will differ among professionals in a nonprocess reality compared to a process reality. For example, it would be incongruent for a physician to ask a nurse for advice or for recommendations about a patient if the physician adopted a nonprocess perspective.

The parameters of that nonprocess relationship would be limited to the physician gathering information from the nurse specific to patient data and concomitantly the nurse would not offer any opinions about care/treatment/diagnoses as s/he recognizes that the physician is in charge and is the identified expert.

The ways that a physician and a nurse with differing reality perspectives relate to each other are realized in a variety of scenarios. For some, an elaborate ritual may be enacted whereby the professional relationship is maintained without any intrusions or loss of discourse. For example, the nurse from a nonprocess perception would not even consider questioning a doctor's order, whereas the aware nurse from a process perspective would not directly question a doctor's order but would cautiously imply that the drug dosage ordered was too high. In this latter instance, an informed player-physician would not take offense and would engage in the pretense of never making a mistake and the player nurse is satisfied that an order was changed without a direct confrontation.[4]

In another instance, a physician may ask for information about a patient. The physician expects facts from the nurse and if the nurse is from a process system s/he may share all kinds of information about the patient, e.g., family, feelings, notions, and subjective data. Soon, the physician from a nonprocess perspective will deliberately select specific nurses to provide the requested patient data. These nurses probably would be nurses from a nonprocess perception or nurses from a process system who learned that nonprocess people usually want facts. The nurse from the latter system would be problematic for the physician if s/he did not change or adopt the desired behavior.

Another area of conflict with the differing systems may be enacted by persons from the two realities in the ways they handle information. One physician may say, "I just feel it, there is still something wrong with the patient even if the test results are negative" whereas a nonprocess physician would ask, "What do feelings have to do with thinking?"

Another source of misunderstandings stems from an unawareness that people construct realities differently. A person who organizes her/his reality with relationships as a focus (process) may ask to weigh a terminally ill patient once a week instead of every third day. Reasons pertaining to the patient's comfort may be given as the rationale for this request. The intent to decrease suffering is the basis for the nurse's request and this stems from the relationship with the patient. The response from someone who constructs a reality with self/work as the center may view the request as simply that the nurse is trying to get out of work or attempting to save herself/himself some time. A solution to the conflicts engendered by an unshared reality is to use the language and adopt the perception of the reality that is contrary to yours. This enables one to function efficiently and effectively. For instance, to enable the patient who is dying to be weighed once a week, it should be demonstrated by facts that changing the weighing schedule would not compromise the treatment/care.

The factors that foster the development of client relationships are often negated as nonscientific. These nurturing modalities are not legitimized or they are viewed as not clinically important. The person who uses nurturing strategies that foster relationships may be viewed as not or less competent nonprocess persons. These strategies are really relationship building that is the basis for the process perception of the world.

Another source of misunderstanding stems from a patient's right to know and the professional's right to act in the patient's best interest. A health professional who adheres to a process reality would support the patient's construction of a personal reality and the philosophy that patients should have the data, that we do not have the right to distort another's reality. However, if a patient distorts his/her own reality, it would follow that one would support that which the patient constructed. In the nonprocess reality, professionals would consider the right to disclosure as theirs alone and would develop various criteria that enabled them to decide when and if disclosure was appropriate. The decision rests totally with the nonprocess professional and s/he is in charge of the information.

IMPLICATIONS

The implications arising from the differing views of reality are several. First, the effort expended in not being wrong fosters the need to be omnipotent. It is unlikely that one can always be omnipotent and always right in the care of patients with incurable illnesses. The patient situations that we are discussing are fraught with uncertainty and ambiguity. There are many junctures at which one can be wrong. Even if one is not wrong, as in the case that a recurrence of cancer and metastasis has a 60 percent probability with surgery, the surgeon may still feel in the wrong. It is a case of being right but feeling wrong. Not to be successful in one's treatment of a patient means that one (i.e., nonprocess system) is a failure or at the very least that one has failed the patient. A process perception would be more supportive of the health professional in no-win situations.

Secondly, there are instances when conclusions about patient care must be reached in an expedient way and the process perspective would greatly hinder or delay decision making. Linear thinking is much more efficient. However, if there is a seemingly unsolvable problem then multidimensional thinking has utility. This latter style of thinking takes more clock time and uses information from a variety of sources, including intuition, thereby allowing for many more possible solutions.

In a nonprocess system, one uses factual data and is more comfortable with certainty and predictability and, in other words, the tenets of the scientific method. In a process system, ambiguity is more easily tolerated. Since in the process system there is an assumption that there are more than two ways of perceiving things, the individual does not have the burden of dualism. S/he can be there for patients and by being there and not necessarily doing anything (i.e., as frequently nothing more can be done) it is enough. Dualism implies that some action is obligatory. In the patient care situations being discussed, it may be in the best interests of the patients to do nothing, e.g., no more surgery, no more chemotherapy, no more heroic methods. In a nonprocess system, to do nothing may be analogous to failing or being wrong and thus the professional encourages the use of one more intervention.

The dominance of any one profession in complex chronic care situations can no longer be any one profession's prerogative. A major shift in the delivery of health care is occurring. No one is totally in control or totally independent of another. The cost of the nonprocess system is that it precludes and limits the integration of all professionals into a team concept. Those persons who exclude themselves from others by virtue of a hierarchical ranking will not have support for their vulnerability, their guilt, their fear of patient and family reactions, and their human limitations in uncontrollable and complex patient situations.

One last implication is that we know very little about the qualitative aspects of chronic and terminal illness. Nurses and social workers are more cognizant than others of some of these dimensions. To engage all health professionals in the care and treatment of patients with chronic and terminal illnesses would greatly enhance the quality of life of patients and their families. To engage all of the team in an interdependent way requires an approach that approximates a process view of the world.

CONCLUSION/RECOMMENDATION

There is usually a lack of awareness that there are different perceptions of reality. There are other possible realities that could be described and classified and the utility of the nonprocess and process realities in understanding health care professionals' relationships is most meritorious.

In the care of the patient who is incurable, the various professionals are faced with the paradox that even if each agreed to who is in charge, none is really in charge or in control or independent of the other. Our lack of knowledge of the other's value system, perceptions of reality, skills, and their contributions hinders the development of any shared realities. For instance, the nurse meets the patient's needs in a qualitatively different way from the approach used by physicians, or by social workers, or by ministers. A nurse's approach or a social worker's approach or a physician's approach is not better, nor is it worse: It is just different. The differences reflect unique capabilities and contributions that could enhance the treatment of any one patient.

To fully appreciate the various contributions from health professions, whether they are from a nonprocess model or a process model, it is suggested that a self-option model be developed. A self-option model would encompass the characteristics of the other models that best enhance patient care and allow for the best from both models.

NOTES*

1. The author initially described the two perspectives of realities as co-operative and competitive and then renamed them to the current terms to maintain some neutrality. It is clear that the words competitive and co-operative have inherent values in connotation.
2. It is hypothesized that the non-process way of considering data occurs in the left brain. The process way is hypothesized to occur in the right brain and data are received from a variety of sources.
3. A surgeon colleague said that he believed that surgeons in the future would need to rely more and more on nurses for information. He said this was a problem as nurses gave so much information that one needs to ferret out what is really important, e.g., factual information.
4. The nurse with a non-process perspective and a physician with a process perspective may engage in the same situation. However, the nurse's intent is to maintain

---

*I gratefully acknowledge the assistance of Barbara Lawton for providing the context that enabled this paper to be completed.

the physician's place in the hierarchal system and not to avoid confrontation. In this situation, both may be frustrated as the physician really works as a team player and not just as someone to unquestioningly accept an order and the nurse isn't satisfied as the physician won't stay in the hierarchical ranking s/he expects.

21

LIFE-THREATENING ILLNESS AND ACTS OF TRUST

PAUL MOORE, JR.

A long history of distrust exists between clergy and doctors based on metaphysical grounds and on territorial imperatives. The gap between us was widest, I would say, in the 1930s and 1940s in the full flower of scientific optimism. Since World War II, the horror of the holocaust and the increasing violence of the world have somehow chastened humanity's confidence in science and has made religion less sure of human progress under a benevolent God. Furthermore, it seems to me that the deeper science probes the physical universe or the human body, the greater grows that which is unknown, the mystery behind empirical data.

So it is that physicians acknowledge areas of agnosticism in their discipline. By the same token, any theologian who is honest, no matter how holy he or she might be, no matter how learned in theology, admits agnosticism about the ultimate nature of God. He or she may have a structured rational system but like the physician, it exists on an hypothesis that cannot be proven. However, in order to function each human being makes some act of faith, conscious or unconscious in order to get up in the morning.

The normal day-to-day living occurs without much questioning of ultimates. However, when death comes near, this dark mysterious void has to be faced, faced by the threatened patient to be sure, but also faced by the family, the doctor, the nurses, and the clergy.

Quite properly, a fear of death exists in us all, but this fear can be healthy or neurotic. It can skew our normal reactions. When my first wife was diagnosed to have cancer, I insisted that the doctor tell her. We had an agreement that there would be no medical secrets between us if either became seriously ill. He opened the conversation thus, "Mrs. Moore, I am sorry I ever met you." He was a first-rate surgeon, a kindly man, but without meaning to, he made a brutally rejecting remark at the very moment the patient needed acceptance. His own self-protection from the fear of death had unconsciously taken over.

The role of the clergyman in these cases is to see and deal with the whole situation, the *whole* cast of characters and the *whole* being—mind, body feeling, spirit—of the patient. He does this as coordinator, interpreter, consultant. The clergyman is a professional. He or she is trained and usually experienced. He often has far more training in the human dynamics of life-threatening situations than does the doctor. Look at it this way. A human being is one person described by a continuum we call body, emotion, mind, spirit. The doctor specializes in the care of the body, unless he or she is a psychiatrist. He is less trained in the emotions, and only by coincidence is he trained in the intellectual and spiritual dimensions of dying. The clergyman, however, is trained in them, perhaps has solid training in psychiatry and only by coincidence, understanding of medicine. Thus, each of us approaches the person at a different point of entry on the continuum and meets the other in the center under the shadow of death.

Now to be more practical as to how the clergyman can assist the doctor: First, he can allay the fear within the patient and family by quiet discussion and prayer. If someone can talk about fear, it ceases to be an unknown monster lurking in the dark. A believer by prayer is able to let go a loved one, to allow God, as it were, to take over. Although most doctors would not admit their need lest it seem like weakness, they cannot help but bear the fear of failure, the loss of face, the awful burden of "telling the family," the decisions of how candid to be, the guilt of not being able to relieve pain. These are subjects the physician can talk over, can unburden to an understanding clergyman. Clergy are at home with death and can talk about it without self-consciousness. They can deal with a patient's ultimate questions, which may go unasked if a clergyman is not there. (Some people have as much trouble talking about death as talking about sex!)

The minister can interpret the doctor to the patient. Many people are afraid of doctors, many become angry at them, many do not understand why certain things are done, many do not comprehend even elementary medical language or are so frightened they cannot hear what the doctor says or refuse to believe either good news or bad. The minister can interpret and reassure, and if necessary inquire for further clarification from the physician.

The decision to end life support systems when recovery of consciousness is medically impossible always is agonizing. Having discussed it intellectually and participated in it pastorally, I was amazed how shaken I was at the prospect of making that decision about my own mother. Thank God, we did not have to. To have a clergyperson present for such a discussion is most salutary, because no matter how obvious the decision seems, guilt and anger are present.

I feel very strongly that withdrawing life support must be a corporate decision. The doctor supplies with care and patience the complete data including financial liability, the clergyman opens up moral and theological considerations, and the family makes the final decision. Even if the family are nonbelievers, it often helps to have a clergyman present because beneath any veneer of skepticism lies a primitive instinctual fear of being a participant in a relative's death.

Finally, most contemporary clergy have some training in the dynamics of death. Most have read in the literature. Thus, they are not surprised at the sometimes bizarre reaction to death.

Most clergy are reasonable human beings. We, of course, like others, have some nuts in our professions too—and we are most grateful when doctors understand and respect our role. By the same token, we attempt to understand and respect the awesome vocation to which they are called.

Part V
RELIEF OF SUFFERING

22

ALTERNATIVE APPROACHES TO THE CONTROL OF PAIN AND DISCOMFORT

Lester C. Mark

The patient suffering pain and discomfort is commonly treated with an appropriate combination of pharmacologic, nerve block, and psychologic technics. Other options include (1) self-hypnosis, (2) bio-feedback, (3) acupuncture, and (4) electric nerve stimulation, applied transcutaneously or via implanted devices.

SELF-HYPNOSIS

Self-hypnosis is a useful technic for the control of pain and discomfort in selected patients. The selection is based on a simple five minute test, the Hypnotic Induction Profile, to identify poorly, moderately, and highly hypnotizable subjects. The test starts with the eye roll sign (Spiegel 1972) which quantifies, on a 0–4 scale, the amount of sclera visible between the lower border of the iris and the lower eyelid as the subject closes the eyes while forcibly looking upward as much as he (or she) can. Next comes hand levitation, the ease with which the hand floats up into the air in response to verbal suggestions that it will do so. Finally, the feeling of disassociation in the levitating hand, the sense of difference in control of that hand compared to the control hand, the number of verbal reinforcements needed to effect the levitation, and any sensations of floating, lightness or heaviness, are all evaluated to contribute to the final score. Assuming an adequate score, the patient can then be instructed in a self-hypnosis exercise designed in accordance with the responses measured and the patient's own wishes.

Hypnotic trance capacity is at its height in young children, most of whom are hypnotizable. Trance capacity declines gradually during adolescence, then remains relatively stable until senescence, when there is a general decline. Two out of three unselected but emotionally stable people are hypnotizable to some degree, while one in ten is highly hypnotizable (Spiegel and Spiegel 1978).

Note that the term itself is a misnomer: hypnosis is not sleep, but a state of focused awareness, of intense concentration on a desired objective. Since all medical hypnosis is self-hypnosis (Spiegel 1981), the motivation is essential. The patient who has learned to use pain for secondary gain, e.g., to manipulate a difficult family situation, to avoid unwanted work, to continue unemployment insurance, will consciously or subconsciously refuse to succeed with self-hypnosis.

The therapist may provide guidance for the patient to learn technics for either (1) general relaxation or (2) specific (pain) therapy.

General relaxation serves as a distraction, directing attention away from the pain to an enjoyable experience, e.g., a beach holiday. The patient is able to ignore discomfort while concentrating on the relaxing sensations.

Specific pain therapy may use imagined heat, cold, numbness, etc., directly in the painful area to ease or obliterate discomfort. So-called "glove anesthesia" experiences the hypnotized hand as filled with Novocaine, numb and heavy. By placing this hand on the skin overlying the painful area, the numbness is enabled to flow into the affected part, thereby effecting the desired analgesia.

Finally, since pain relief whose duration is restricted to the actual period of trance (and ends when the patient emerges from the trance state) is of limited usefulness, instruction is offered in use of the post-hypnotic suggestion, whereby discomfort and subjective well-being are enabled to persist beyond the formal trance. The usefulness of hypnosis to control pain or other symptoms is limited only by the capability and motivation of the patient and the skill and ingenuity of the therapist. The encouragement and support of nursing and other personnel can be most helpful.

BIOFEEDBACK

Biofeedback training utilizes electronic instrumentation capable of visual and/or auditory displays to provide moment-to-moment data concerning physiologic phenomena, e.g., skin temperature, electro-myographic (EMG) activity, pulse rate, not ordinarily deemed subject to voluntary control (Greenspan 1981). The information enables the individual, in a series of trial-and-error learning sessions, to establish volitional control over the selected function. For example, a patient with Raynaud's disease, suffering the pain of peripheral vasospasm, may discover in his first biofeedback session that the temperature of his hands fluctuates and that he can warm them 2–3°F, a change too subtle to alter his pain. Nevertheless, the information allows him to proceed along a learning curve which will eventually result in pain reduction. Over the course of several training sessions, he begins to reexperience the internal responses that accompany the warming, until the changes are large enough to be appreciated as diminished pain (Greenspan 1981).

Each biofeedback session should begin with a period of guided relaxation. Eyes closed, the patient is helped to shift mental gears by breathing deeply and slowly, and alternately tensing and relaxing each group of muscles in turn, from toes to scalp. Thus, eliminating physical and emotional tension heightens the patient's ability to focus on the information chosen for the biofeedback training.

The sessions help the adult to learn innate but previously unavailable responses to stress and pain, much as a young child learns to master basic motor and autonomic functions. The therapeutic sessions include appropriate reinforcements and support for the patient from the biofeedback training, much as the parent provides for the learning child. Each process assumes that self-mastery is both feasible and desirable.

The practicability of biofeedback technics to control pain is illustrated in a series of 11 patients with peripheral vascular disease (Greenspan et al. 1980). None could walk as much as 0.2 mile on a treadmill (set at 10 percent incline, 2¼ mph) without suffering the pain of intermittent claudication. EMG feedback from the frontalis muscle and skin temperature feedback from hands and feet were provided in 3 sessions weekly for 13 weeks, after which 7 of 11 patients could walk either 30 minutes or more than a mile without pain. All patients in the treatment group improved beyond the slight improvement attributable to a learning effect, shown by the controls ($P < 0.01$) (Greenspan et al. 1980). Comparison of brachial to ankle blood pressures obtained before and after treadmill walking showed decreased peripheral vascular resistance to the leg, not only immediately after the course of therapy but also 3, 6, and 12 months later.

Other applications of this approach combining biofeedback and relaxation therapy include Raynaud's disease (Jackson et al. 1973; May and Weber 1976), tension (Budyneski et al. 1973; Cox, Freundlich, and Myer 1975; Hutchings and Reinking 1976) and migraine (Sargent, Green, and Walters 1973; Turin and Johnson 1976) headaches, low back pain (Greenspan 1981) and dysmenorrhea. In all instances, home practice reinforces the beneficial effects of training in the laboratory.

ACUPUNCTURE

Acupuncture, perhaps the most maligned therapy since hypnosis, is gradually achieving a role in the area of pain management. This is partially due to the emergence of scientific rationale in the forms of the gate control theory of pain suppression (Melzack and Wall 1965) and the discovery that acupuncture causes release of beta-endorphin, ACTH and serotonin in the CNS (Han and Terenius 1982) and partly to increased acceptance and usage by respectable medical practitioners. The technic is most useful for patients with musculoskeletal disorders, e.g., osteoarthritis, rheumatoid arthritis, low back pain, cervical radiculopathy, cephalalgia, temporomandibular and other dental pains, especially when more usual treatment modalities prove unsuccessful (Bannerman 1980). Indeed, since it is simple, painless, and relatively innocuous, acupuncture merits trial in instances of failure of conventional therapy or in cases of drug intolerance, e.g., allergic or sensitivity reactions, peptic ulcer, etc. (Lee 1981). Fine (28–32 or smaller gauge) needles are inserted at appropriate points, where they remain quietly in situ or are stimulated manually, electrically, or (in the People's Republic of China) thermally (Mark 1981). Treatments lasting up to 20–30 minutes may be administered initially twice weekly, then weekly. Favorable responses occur in 50 percent of patients within 3 treatments, and in 90–95 percent within 6 (Lee 1981). Hyperemia, frequently noted at the site of insertion of the needle and attributed to release of histamine-like substances (Omura 1975), is a good prognosis sign (Lee 1981).

Criteria of efficacy of acupuncture therapy include reduction in pain medication, increases in muscle strength and in range of motion of painful joints, and functional improvement in performing daily tasks

(Lee 1981). Concomitant therapy, e.g., massage, heat, exercise, can be helpful.

Hazards and precautions (Lee 1981; Carron, Epstein, and Grand 1974) include syncope (new patients should recline during initial therapy), hematoma formation (as with nerve blocks and injection therapy, acupuncture needling is contraindicated in the presence of disorders of blood clotting), pneumothorax (especially with needling in the base of the neck or over the apex of the lung), and injury to other vital organs (due to injudiciously deep needling; knowledge of anatomy is essential!). Aseptic technic, with properly sterilized needles (disposable ones are now available) and skin cleansing (with alcohol or other antiseptic agents) are mandatory. Needles should obviously not be inserted through areas of inflammation, psoriasis, herpes, or malignancy. Strong stimulation of needles should be avoided in pregnant or epileptic individuals, and patients with cardiac or diaphragmatic pacemakers should not receive electroacupuncture.

ELECTRIC NERVE STIMULATION

Neurostimulation applied transcutaneously or via implanted devices to various parts of the nervous system offers yet another alternative for pain control. Like acupuncture, the results are explainable in terms of the gate control theory, endogenous opiates, or serotonin (Ray 1980).

Transcutaneous electric nerve stimulation (TENS) is so simple and so lacking in side effects (except for occasional unpleasant tingling sensations or muscle contractions) that it merits trial in almost any instance of circumscribed pain (Ray 1981). The stimuli are applied via surface electrodes, generally placed adjacent to the site of pain or over a nearby sensory nerve, but the best location should be sought in each patient. The stimulating devices themselves offer a variety of parameters to adjust, including frequency, intensity, and configuration, but despite frequent references to "preferred" stimulus wave forms, there appear to be none (Ray 1981). Indeed, it seems more important that the stimulation be reasonably comfortable.

TENS therapy has been successfully applied to a variety of body surface locations (often coinciding with established acupuncture points) (Melzack, Stillwell, and Fox 1977), e.g., the head (for headache, temporomandibular joint syndrome, dental pain, sinusitis, occipital neuralgia), neck, shoulder, upper and lower back and extremities, to phantom limbs and even to postoperative wound pain (Ray 1981).

Other devices are available for implantation for peripheral nerve neurostimulation (PNS or PNN), stimulation of spinal cord, either via percutaneously implanted spinal cord epidural stimulation (PISCES) or via operatively placed devices for dorsal column neurostimulation (DCN) or deep brain stimulation (DBS).

PNS implants are useful for pain in one limb distal to the implant, usually on the ulnar nerve or brachial plexus (Campbell and Long 1976).

The PISCES or PENS (percutaneous epidural nerve stimulation) systems are most suitable if at least 60 percent if the pain is located in one limb, but has also been useful in "failed back surgery" (Ray 1981). Other applications, often with dramatic results, include phantom limb pain, partial denervation states, diabetic neuropathy and posttraumatic pain (Burton, Ray, and Nashold 1977). The electrodes are inserted under X-ray image intensifier control through two guide needles into the epidural space, and the best locations determined by intraoperative stimulation. Final placement depends upon the pain response and the subjective sensation of stimulation (Ray 1981) verified over the next few days.

The DCN implantation is more formidable since it requires a laminectomy to permit placement of the electrodes within layers of dura, rather than subdural or subarachnoid, to reduce the likelihood of fibrosis (and decreased efficacy) (Ray 1981). DBS implants, the last resort, may be the most effective stimulation technic to control severe, agonizing, unremitting pain, especially bilateral, deep, midline or diffuse chronic pain, pain due to metastatic cancer (if life expectancy is sufficiently long), or recurrent pain after ablative operations on the CNS intended to control a difficult pain problem. The target areas are (1) the periaqueductal gray or paraventricular complex for deep-seated pain or (2) the specific sensory thalamus or medial lemniscus for superficial or deafferentation pain (Ray 1981). Side effects of eye movements, hypertension, anxiety or headache may be minimized by careful adjustment of the stimulation.

Note that all forms of neurostimulators are characterized by being nonaddicting, under direct patient control, and causing no undesirable side effects that cannot be eliminated by reducing or stopping the stimulation.

REFERENCES

Bannerman, R.H. 1980. "The World Health Organization Viewpoint on Acupuncture." *American Journal of Acupuncture* 8:213–235.

Budyneski, T.H., J.M. Stoyva, C.S. Adler, and D.J. Mullaney. 1973. "EMG Biofeedback and Tension Headache: A Controlled Outcome Study." *Psychosomatic Medicine* 35:484–496.

Burton, C.V., C.D. Ray, and B.S. Nashold, eds., 1977. "Symposium on the Safety and Clinical Efficacy of Implanted Neuroaugmentive Devices." *Neurosurgery* 1:185–232.

Campbell, J.N. and D.M. Long. 1976. "Peripheral Nerve Stimulation in the Treatment of Intractable Pain." *Journal of Neurological Surgery* 45:692–699.

Carron, H., B.S. Epstein, and B. Grand. 1974. "Complications of Acupuncture." *Journal of the American Medical Association* 228:1552–1554.

Cox, D.J., A. Freundlich, and R.G. Myer. 1975. "Differential Effectiveness of Electromyogram Feedback Treatment for Muscle Contraction Headache." *Consultations in Clinical Psychology* 43:892–899.

Greenspan, K. 1981. "Biofeedback in the Control of Chronic Pain." In L.C. Mark, ed., *Pain Control: Practical Aspects of Patient Care*, New York: Masson.

Greenspan, K., P. Lawrence, A. Voorhees, and D. Esposito. 1980. "The Role of Biofeedback and Relaxation Therapy in Arterial Occlusive Disease." *Journal of Surgical Research* 29:387–394.

Han, J.S. and L. Terenius. 1982. "Neurochemical Basis of Acupuncture and Analgesia." *Annual Review of Pharmacology and Toxicology* 22:193–220.

Hutchings, D.R. and R.H. Reinking. 1976. "Tension Headaches: What Form of Therapy Is Most Effective?" *Biofeedback and Self Regulation* 1:183–190.

Jacobson, A.M., T.P. Hackett, O.S. Surman, and E.L. Silverberg. 1973. "Raynaud's Phenomenon: Treatment with Hypnotic Operant Technique." *Journal of the American Medical Association* 225:739–740.

Lee, M.H.M. 1981. "Acupuncture for Pain Control." In L.C. Mark, ed., *Pain Control: Practical Aspects of Patient Care*, New York: Masson.

Mark, L.C. 1981. "Observations on Pain Control in the People's Republic of China. In L.C. Mark, ed., *Pain Control: Practical Aspects of Patient Care*, New York: Masson.

May, D.S. and C.A. Weber. 1976. "Temperature Feedback Training with Symptom Reduction in Raynaud's Disease: A Controlled Study." Presented at the 7th Annual Meeting, Biofeedback Research Society, Colorado Springs, February.

Melzack, R., D. Stillwell, and E. Fox. 1977. "Trigger Points and Acupuncture Points for Pain: Correlations and Implications." *Pain* 3:23.

Melzack, R. and P. Wall. 1965. "Pain Mechanisms: A New Theory." *Science* 150:971–979.

Morgan, A.H. and E.R. Hilgard. 1973. "Age Differences in Susceptibility to Hypnosis." *International Journal of Clinical and Experimental Hypnosis* 21:78–85.

Omura, Y. 1975. "Patho-physiology of Acupuncture Treatment: Effects of Acupuncture on Cardiovascular and Nervous Systems." *Acupuncture and Electrotherapeutic Research* 1:51–140.

Ray, C.D. 1981. "Spinal Epidural Electrical Stimulation for Pain Control: Practical Details and Results." *Applied Neurophysiology* 44:194–206.

Ray, C.D. 1981. "Neurostimulation for Control of Pain." In L.C. Mark, ed., *Pain Control: Practical Aspects of Patient Care*, New York: Masson.

Sargent, J.D., E.E. Green, and E.D. Walters. 1973. "Preliminary Report on the Use of Autogenic Feedback Training in the Treatment of Migraine and Tension Headache." *Psychosomatic Medicine* 35:2,129.

Spiegel, D. 1981. "Self-Hypnosis in the Management of Chronic Pain." In L.C. Mark, ed., *Pain Control: Practical Aspects of Patient Care*, New York: Masson.

Spiegel, H. 1972. "An Eye-Roll Test for Hypnotizability." *American Journal of Clinical Hypnosis* 15:25–28.

Spiegel, H. and D. Spiegel. 1978. *Trance and Treatment: Clinical Uses of Hypnosis.* New York: Basic Books.

Turin, A. and W.G. Johnson. 1976. "Biofeedback Therapy for Migraine Headaches." *Archives of General Psychiatry* 33:517.

23

THE SURGEON'S ROLE IN PROVIDING PALLIATIVE TREATMENT OF THE CANCER PATIENT

PAUL LoGERFO

Surgery is still the main and often the only curative form of treatment for most cancers. Usually, the surgeon is central figure in the treatment of many malignant diseases. As some cancers become more responsive to new and better forms of chemotherapy, however, this situation may be gradually changing. Although great satisfaction is derived from curing cancer by surgery, the real test of a surgeon's skill and experience comes in dealing with patients who have incurable disease. The surgeon who takes on the care of a patient with early cancer must be willing to accept the potential responsibility of caring for patients with terminal disease. The extent of the commitment may not be apparent initially when the prognosis seems bright, but recurrences must be looked for in all patients and when they occur the extent of the surgeon's commitment becomes more apparent.

When a patient is first evaluated for malignant disease, it is important to explain the tests that will be necessary and the alternatives available. The possibility of cancer and/or other diseases should be confronted at that time. It is surprising how often breaking the emotional barrier associated with the word "cancer" can open communication and allow patients to express their fears and anxieties. If surgery is anticipated, it is useful to discuss the possibility of an incurable situation prior to the operation since it is not uncommon to find that the operation is only

149

palliative. It is also often advisable to tell the patient that a combination of chemotherapy and/or radiotherapy in addition to surgery might be the recommended treatment for the disease. The patient should be informed that the decision regarding such modalities will be based on the exact type of cancer and on the surgical findings at the time of operation. Although some might argue that this kind of discussion may be deceptive to the patient with newly diagnosed cancer, it has the effect of giving the patient confidence that the physician is anticipating all possibilities and decreases the fears associated with changes in therapy. There is no question that explaining an incurable situation to a patient is always difficult despite whatever preoperative preparation may have been carried out. The negative connotations associated with the words "incurable cancer" are almost insurmountable. Despite the efforts of many people and organizations to decrease the fears associated with this diagnosis, the experience of most people who deal with this on a day-to-day basis is that the fear is truly justified.

When patients are sent to a surgeon with a diagnosis of incurable cancer based on another physician's assessment, it is advisable to review the information thoroughly. Aggressive therapy might cure or provide palliation that may not only prolong life but also might greatly improve its quality. Modalities of therapy change and often what might seem to be curable to well-trained oncologists might be overlooked by the less experienced. Equally devastating to the patient is the surgeon who believes that any treatment is better than doing nothing and is not able to face realistically the limitations of treatment. Patients caught in this situation are often given new hope and can become victims of unnecessary surgery. It is not uncommon to have a patient with incurable disease who has been told by an experienced surgeon that his situation is best treated by nonoperative means. Patients will often seek the opinions of many surgeons and will eventually find someone who will be willing to operate on them. These surgeons offer hope to desperate patients but are really only interested in a technical exercise, and their motivation must be seriously questioned. It is surprising how often surgeons and institutions have become famous by taking on hopeless patients whom any well trained surgical oncologist would recognize as incurable.

Advising terminal cancer patients of their diagnosis and prognosis is difficult. The method in which each patient is told is highly individualistic. Some patients, having been informed of their diagnosis, will deliberately evade all further disclosures about their disease but will continue to accept treatment in a trusting manner. I believe, however, that to deny the patient the truth is unsatisfactory and that most people can be told and indeed want to be told. A meaningful trusting relationship conducive to providing optimal care cannot be established without a clear understanding of what the problem is. How the truth is told, however, is an art that is easily acquired by some but, unfortunately, not by all. Sometimes other physicians and health providers interfere with developing this dialogue by evading the issue, implying that what was told was not as bad as it may seem. When patients are told several different stories by different physicians, it is often confusing to them. Therefore, it is important that all physicians involved in the case clearly understand what the patient has been told so that they can answer questions in a consistent and constructive manner.

Any discussion of the diagnosis with a relatively healthy patient who has just undergone palliative surgery is best done initially with the patient alone. As soon as it is reasonably convenient, a discussion of planned treatments with both the patient and the closest family member is important. This breaks down barriers in communication between patients and the ones closest to them. It is important to eliminate the burden of game playing between family members by having open discussions. In many instances, family members try to get the physician aside to hear—they think—something that cannot be told to the patient. Depending on the situation, I often handle such problems by bringing the family member back into the patient's room and then repeating the question in a constructive way so that the patient does not think secrets are being kept from him. In addition, it gives patients assurance that they do have some control over their lives. Regardless of how the situation is handled, when an incurable cancer is found, the role of the surgeon changes from that of a curer to a reliever of pain and anguish. The surgeon often becomes a concerned advisor who guides further treatment, whether it be chemotherapy, radiation therapy, or a combination of different modalities.

There are no easy ways to extend life without paying some price. For each individual the value of the treatment is different when measured against what he considers a meaningful existence. The aged patient who feels totally fulfilled might not be as willing to accept the difficulties of treatment as a young parent. Each form of medical treatment—surgery, chemotherapy, and radiation therapy—carries its own benefits, risks, and disadvantages. It is the physician's responsibility to guide the patient through alternatives and select the therapy that fits in with the individual patient's best interests. Balancing of the disadvantages against the quality of life gained requires judgment that usually comes only with experience. In the early phases of terminal disease, the recommendations of individual physicians are fairly consistent, but decisions often become a matter of controversy in the later phases of the disease because the experiences and values of different physicians in dealing with dying patients may not be the same. In dealing with oncological problems, differences are greatly decreased as the experiences of the physicians dealing with cancer increase. The treatment recommendations made by a group of medical oncologists, surgeons, and radiation therapists will be more in agreement if they are all 50 than if they are all 35, particularly concerning the end phase of the disease. The guiding principle in all decisions should be to delay anguish and suffering, and to extend a life whose quality is satisfactory to the individual.

The indication of surgical treatment of patients with terminal illness does not differ greatly from treatment to the patient with a nonterminal disease. But the problem lies in who should get the treatment. Clearly, the cachectic patient who presents with an abdominal emergency in the late phase of disease has little to gain from surgical intervention. Those who benefit most are those diagnosed in the early phases of an incurable illness that is not associated with extensive systemic and/or organ failure. The time between the initial documentation of incurability and the terminal phases of the disease has been referred to as the period of grace. During this period, surgical procedures may be undertaken without great risk and the patient will clearly show improvement after recovery from surgery to the extent that a relatively normal life can be resumed. In many instances, surgical therapy is accepted by the patient with an optimistic attitude that all is not so bad. These procedures are usually elective, although some of them may be placed in the nonelective category such as in the case of intestinal obstruction. When reviewing survival statistics of palliative surgical operations in people with gastrointestinal cancers, the amount of life gained by operative intervention is only measured in months although the quality of remaining life may be greatly improved. This improvement is short-lived in most patients, but there are always some patients who thrive after palliative procedures. The surgeon who believes palliative surgery always pays dividends is clearly not very observant. Yet it is difficult for any of us to make judgments on available statistics since there are patients with slow growing cancers who lead a relatively normal existence for long periods of time after their palliative surgery. Some patients outlive the norm. They provide hope for any individual facing palliative surgery and the surgeon who has cared for one of these exceptional patients will continue to advise palliative procedures for others. Surgical selection is still paramount to assuring reasonable results and this is largely dependent on surgical judgment. Clearly, some patients with short survivals should have been advised not to have surgery by their physician. The main goal of palliative surgery is to relieve pain and suffering while prolonging a comfortable extension of life.

Some surgical procedures are gradually being replaced by less invasive forms of therapy such as biliary drainage, or nephrostomy tubes placed percutaneously by the radiologist. These procedures prevent an immense amount of pain and suffering and have a high benefit to cost ratio for the patient. Their main disadvantage is that they leave patients with external drainage tubes. Many surgeons feel that the quality of life is decreased by these procedures. Obviously, the decision to elect their procedures remains a highly personal one. Yet, radiological procedures, along with effective chemotherapy and radiotherapy, are welcomed by the physician who knows the limits of surgery.

Superficial tumors involving the integument may bleed, become infected, and ulcerate. Sometimes they may be aesthetically unpleasing and often malodorous. Surgical removal of these lesions, some of which are extremely slow growing, may add considerably to the quality of life.

The delivery of chemotherapy via arterial or venous fusion systems by implantable pumps or closed perfusion techniques is sometimes useful in patients with metastatic disease. Perfusion of extremities in malignant melanoma or sarcoma is a well accepted form of therapy which is useful, but only in a limited number of patients. Endocrine manipulations such as oophectomy or adrenalectomy have been shown to be useful in the treatment of breast cancer, but these surgical procedures have been largely replaced by medical therapy. Prostatic cancer still is effectively treated by castration. These are some of the ways that surgery can benefit the incurable patient in the early phase of the disease. Once the disease has progressed to the point where vital organ systems begin to fail, then aggressive palliative surgery is fruitless and will only increase the suffering and hasten the patient's demise. Then, the physician's main efforts must be directed toward measures that will provide emotional support and comfort. Hopefully, the patient can be cared for in an environment which maintains dignity while allowing some self control—if not at home as close to it as possible. Making family members feel comfortable while caring for a terminally ill loved one is the goal that most of us strive for. A problem often encountered in a late phase of disease is the acute surgical emergency in a patient who has received extensive chemotherapy and/or radiation. If the patient is unknown to the surgeon, the decision about operation is often based on his prior judgment in treating surgical emergencies in nonmalignant disease. The surgeon's first instinct is an aggressive one, for surgical therapy will often totally cure a patient with nonmalignant disease. For the patient who is in the late phases of a malignant disease, aggressive surgical therapy is often disastrous. I have recently had the opportunity to review a group of 18 patients presenting in this situation. Only three patients left the hospital and the maximum survival time was 3.5 months. Clearly, this may be interpreted as overtreatment, but a common scenario in all these people was that there was no single identifiable physician in charge who had a close relationship with the patient. Having a previously involved physician on call is, I believe, the single most important thing in making the right decisions for each individual situation.

It is not possible to outline an exact plan of treatment for all incurable patients since cancer is very variable and each individual's needs and attitudes can differ in small but important ways. But helping these who are dying is a noble goal that makes death more a part of living for everyone involved.

24

UREMIA—A WAY OUT

Harris M. Nagler

Renal failure may be due to glomerulonephritis, diabetic nephropathy, drug abuse or a multitude of other etiologies. However, each of these etiologies has in common the fact that the *primary* morbid process is the renal failure. In another population of patients, renal failure is secondary to a "more malignant" process. This population is made up of patients who are dying of malignancies of the bladder, prostate, uterus, cervix or any other pelvic viscera in which secondary obstruction of the urinary tract occurs resulting in renal failure. The age distribution of these patients is similar to the incidence of cancer in the population at large. It is this group of patients that may be overlooked in the discussion of the thanatologic aspects of end stage renal disease. Although the emphasis for dialysis and transplant patients is on living with end stage renal disease, for other patients, dying of end stage renal disease may be preferable to dying from their primary, more painful malignant process.

Renal failure secondary to malignancy is due to bilateral ureteral obstruction. The presentation of this may be signs of azotemia, sepsis, and anuria or pain. The timing of this presentation in the patient's history of carcinoma can be quite variable. Bilateral ureteral obstruction may be the initial manifestation of a pelvic malignancy or it may be the result of a malignancy whose presence has been known for many years.

Various primary malignancies may cause bilateral ureteral obstruction. The most common malignancy leading to bilateral ureteral obstruction is that of bladder carcinoma. In three large series, bladder carcinoma accounted for greater than 20 percent of the cases (Holden, McPhee, and

155

Grabstalde 1979; Brin, Schiff, and Weiss 1975; Sharer, Grayhack, and Graham 1978). Carcinoma of the cervix is the next leading offender in terms of malignancies leading to ureteral obstruction. Prostatic carcinoma accounts for between 5 and 15 percent and gastrointestinal carcinoma account for between 10 and 20 percent of azotemic secondary ureteral obstructions. There are other miscellaneous tumors that also lead to ureteral obstruction.

We have been taught that the excellent medical care that we strive to achieve is based on aggressive investigation and aggressive therapy. Certainly, this is a reasonable foundation on which to base the practice of medicine. However, one has to keep in mind certain basic tenets when dealing with patients with malignancies. Our primary objective is to cure patients when possible. When this is not possible, we aim to prolong life as well as to improve the quality of that life. Although when practiced individually these tenets are admirable and achievable, practiced together they may at times conflict. Bilateral ureteral obstruction, renal failure, and advanced malignancy in a patient may make it impossible for the physician to fulfill these basic goals of treatment. Prolonging life through advanced technology in such a situation may diminish the quality of that life.

The synthesis of these goals is to return the patient to a "useful" life (Holden, McPhee, and Grabstalde 1979). This term is tainted with subjective and perhaps distasteful judgmental overtones, but the intent of this terminology is good. The patient should be comfortable and without severe pain. The patient should not be subjected to a series of surgical procedures, one after the other with no end in sight. The patient should be continent and dry. The patient should have the ability to be aware of what he or she is experiencing, and ideally, the patient should be able to be discharged from the hospital. In order to achieve these goals, the patient with bilateral renal obstruction will require intervention or otherwise die in renal failure.

Death from renal failure or azotemia may be relatively painless and comfortable for the patient, whereas, if the progression of renal failure is halted and progression of cancer continues, the death awaiting the patient will be painful. At times, renal obstruction will present with a calamity, such as pain or urosepsis. In these situations, the goal is improved symptom control, and some sort of urinary diversion must be carried out for acute palliation. In an acute crisis situation, this must be offered.

In other patients, renal failure secondary to bilateral ureteral obstruction may have a more insidious onset. The patient may present with symptoms of azotemia. If the neoplasm leading to the obstruction is otherwise stable, or treatable, diversion is generally carried out. If there is potential for independent existence or if the quality of life as a result from the urinary diversion is acceptable, diversion of some sort is carried out.

The decision for therapy or diversion is difficult. It can only be made after weighing the attendant morbidity, the probability of a response, the expected duration of the response, and the availability of as yet unutilized therapies.

There are some relative contraindications to urinary diversion. Patients whose malignancy has progressed to a degree that pain is no longer responsive to medical management; patients who have had a continued downward course in spite of having had all therapeutic modalities may indeed not be patients who would be benefited by urinary diversion. However, the only absolute contraindication is the patient who is unwilling to undergo a procedure which will prolong a progressive, downward course. Whenever possible, it is the patient who should decide whether or not urinary diversion is attempted.

Urinary diversion takes many forms. The classical nephrostomy in which a tube is placed in the kidney has brought urinary diversion into much disfavor. The complication rate is significant. Patients often require several procedures, and still never leave the hospital. In a large series of 218 patients, 45 percent of the patients had major complications after formal nephrostomy (Holden, McPhee, Grabstalde 1979). Thirty-five percent had genitourinary sepsis. When urinary diversion by nephrostomy was carried in patients with Stage A disease, meaning tumors confined or localized to the organ of origin, 100 percent of the patients were afforded "useful" life as described above. Of patients with Stage B tumors, or tumors with local extension or regional metastases, only 40 percent were afforded a useful life; of patients who had widespread metastatic Stage C and D disease, only 27 percent were afforded a useful life for two months from the time of urinary diversion.

Of patients with Stage B disease, 32 percent were dead within two months and 49 percent of patients with Stage C disease were dead within two months. The majority of patients in the categories C and D were unable to leave the hospital after their urinary diversion. One has to question the quality of life afforded these patients as indicated by an objective definition.

Recent advances have supplanted formal nephrostomy placement with internal urinary diversionary techniques. These techniques allow one to bypass the point of urinary obstruction and permit the kidney to drain into the urinary bladder. This has the advantage of avoiding an external urinary appliance as well as avoiding a formal surgical operative procedure for placement of the nephrostomy. Internal urinary diversion dates back to the 1960s when Zimskind developed an indwelling silicone stent which passed from the kidney down to the bladder. This, however, tended to migrate out through the ureter (Zimskind, Fetter, and Wilkerson 1970). There were several developments over the ensuing decade but it was not until 1976 that a reliable, easily placed, indwelling ureteral catheter was developed (Hepperlen and Mardis 1976). This is referred to as a pigtail ureteral catheter in which there is a curlicue pigtail at the proximal ends, preventing migration of the catheter downward and maintaining its ability to divert the urinary flow through an otherwise obstructed ureter. Subsequent modification added a J at both proximal and distal ends which prevented migration in either direction (Finney 1978). These catheters can be placed either in a retrograde fashion endoscopically via the bladder or through a nephrostomy tube placed percutaneously through the flank (Smith et al. 1978; Bigongiari et al. 1980). Either procedure may be performed under local anesthesia. These techniques have the advantage of potentially avoiding a general anesthesia and, more importantly, avoiding the need for external urinary collection devices. As a result of being "internalized," there is no possibility for dislodgement or leakage around the catheter, both complications having in the past been the source of significant problems for patients with formal nephrostomies.

Indwelling, internal ureteral stents eliminate many of the problems that previously plagued patients with formal nephrostomy. Although the period of follow-up for this relatively new technique is short, preliminary studies seem to indicate that the quality of the life afforded these patients is significantly better (Finney 1978; Hepperlen 1979). The major problem with a nephrostomy, as indicated above, is urosepsis (Holden, McPhee, and Grabstalde 1979). Internal diversionary technique largely eliminates the operative complications of nephrostomy requiring general anesthesia. The poor quality of life resulting from external urinary drainage with leakage, dislodgement, sepsis, and the repetitive procedures that often accompany a formal nephrostomy are similarly avoided by internal diversionary techniques. Although the technique is relatively new and the follow-up is of short duration, preliminary results indicate that the time spent in the hospital utilizing internal diversionary techniques is significantly less as compared to patients who underwent formal nephrostomies (Finney 1978; Hepperlen, Mardis, and Kammandel 1979). Of patients with Stage B disease, 4 percent of their remaining life was spent in the hospital; whereas of patients with Stage C disease, 11 percent of their remaining life was spent in the hospital. This compares favorably with the results reported with a nephrostomy tube drainage in which after diversion approximately ⅔ of the patients' survival time was spent in the hospital.

After the decision has been made with the patient to proceed with urinary diversion for malignant ureteral obstruction, the approach should follow the outlined pattern. Attempts at catheterization of the ureter should be carried out endoscopically. When possible, stents should be placed to afford internal urinary diversion. If this fails, a percutaneous nephrostomy may be placed and this may subsequently be converted into an internalized urinary diversionary technique using double J ureteral catheter. If not, this may remain externalized to a collection bag. This is not the most desirable result because some of the same complications of formal nephrostomies will occur. Prior to proceeding with attempts at internal urinary diversion, the patient must be aware that the result may be an externalized urinary diversion.

Technically, we have made great advances in our ability to afford comfortable urinary diversion to patients with malignant ureteral obstruction. However, the capacity to act does not in itself justify the action. The need to treat because we were trained to prolong life and because we are capable of prolonging life is no longer acceptable. The patient, the quality of life, and the dignity of life and of death must be taken into consideration before a urinary diversion should be offered to those with progressive carcinoma that has not responded to other available therapies. Indeed, renal failure may offer a painless, peaceful demise to a patient who might otherwise be subjected to a tormenting death.

REFERENCES

Bigongiari, L. R. et al. 1980. "Conversion of Percutaneous Ureteral Stent to Indwelling Pigtail Stent Over Guidewire." *Urology* XV 5: 461–465.

Brin, E. N., M. Schiff, Jr., and R. M. Weiss. 1975. "Palliative Urinary Diversion for Pelvic Malignancy." *Journal of Urology* 113: 619.

Finney, R. P. 1978. "Experience with New Double J Ureteral Catheter Stent." *Journal of Urology* 120: 678–681.

Hepperlen, T. K. and H. K. Mardis. 1976. "Pigtail Stent Termed Means of Lessening Ureteral Surgery." *Clinical Trends in Urology* 4 & 5.

Hepperlen, T. K. and H. K. Mardis. 1977. "Self Retaining Stent Is Termed Ideal." *Clinical Trends in Urology* 5: 1.

Hepperlen, T. W., H. K. Mardis, and H. Kammandel. 1979. "The Pigtail Ureteral Stent in the Cancer Patient." *Journal of Urology* 121: 17–21.

Holden, S., M. McPhee, and H. Grabstalde. 1979. "The Rationale of Urinary Diversion in Cancer Patients." *Journal of Urology* 121: 19–21.

Part VI
ETHICAL AND MORAL DILEMMAS IN CAREGIVING DECISIONS

25

CLINICAL DECISION MAKING: AN ASSUMED ART

Harold M. Schoolman

Problem solving is the activity of physicians which makes them indispensible in patient care. Problem solving may be thought of as sequential decision making, but our concern here may be narrowed even further, for our interest is in decision making in the face of uncertainty. For rational men, uncertainty tends to provoke anxiety. Yet our concern is not primarily with how the physician deals with his own anxiety when making decisions in the presence of uncertainty but rather how he assures that those decisions are designed for his patient's benefit. To summarize then, we are concerned with the role of the physician in clinical decision making in the face of anxiety provoking uncertainty acting as a patient advocate. To discharge this responsibility, the doctor must make assessments that are based on his appreciation of the changing interactions between the patient, his environment and his disease. I shall not dwell on how we educate physicians to accomplish this difficult task. In general, we assume that like a contagious disease, given sufficient exposure, they will contract the art.

The more pertinent question is how successful are we at such problem solving? Can we rely on this assumed art and is there indeed a scientific basis of this art?

To attempt to gain some insight into these questions we might start with methods of dealing with uncertainty in medicine. For the purpose of this discussion we define uncertainty in terms of probability and for probability use the mathematical definition of relative frequency. We recognize that uncertainty is inherent in the biologic system with which we deal and cannot be eliminated. We choose, therefore, to find a method for measuring it. Thus, for more than half a century medicine has been actively involved in trying to incorporate statistical inference into clinical decision making. That this effort has not been entirely successful can be best understood by recognizing certain intrinsic conflicts in the perspectives of the statistician and the clinician. The first is, perhaps, psychological and was well stated by the editor of *Lancet* in 1937 when in introducing a series of papers by Sir Austin Bradford Hill, he wrote:

> They afford one of the few examples in which the use, or abuse, of mathematical methods tends to induce a strong emotional reaction in non-mathematical minds. This is because statisticians apply to problems, in which we are interested, a technique we do not understand. It is exasperating when we have studied a problem by methods we have spent laborious years in mastering, to find our conclusions questioned and perhaps refuted by someone who could not have made the observations himself. It requires more equanimity than most of us possess to acknowledge that the fault is in ourselves.

Whether or not we understand these methods, there has been an enormous increase in the use of statistical methods and statistical inference in medicine since those words were written. Moreover, a large number of authors' conclusions in published papers are predicated on their interpretation of statistical inference. In a moment we will have a closer look at that use of statistical methods. But first, what is meant by statistical inference and what is its relationship to probability?

Probability is, of course, a branch of mathematics like geometry or algebra. It states that given a distribution and the parameters that characterize it one can find a unique answer to the question, what is the probability (relative frequency) of any outcome in that distribution? For example, given a "normal" or Gaussian distribution of a continuous variable such as height or diastolic blood pressure and the parameters mean (u) and standard deviation (6) which characterize it, one can state that a value between u $\pm$ 6 will occur 67 percent of the time. There is a straightforward and unique answer. Statistics, on the other hand, say given a sample of N observations from a distribution we will presume to know (e.g., normal or Gaussian) what can we infer about the parameters u and 6? Clearly, there is no unique answer. To help the inference process and to put it in the more familiar form, let us take two (or more) samples and assume they are taken from the same distribution (null hypothesis). Then the mean of each sample will be an estimate of the parameter u, the mean of the population, and the difference between the two means, since each is an estimate of the same u, should be zero whatever u may be. The standard deviation of each sample is also an estimate of the standard deviation of the population 6, so the average of the two estimates must be the best available estimate of 6. Without worrying about the niceties we can say that the two sample means if drawn from the same population would differ from each other by 2 or more standard deviations only 5 percent of the time. Therefore, if the two sample means do differ by more than 26, we reject the hypothesis that they are both samples from the same population. In any given experiment, of course, we never know whether the two samples are from the same population. However, if we keep playing the game according to these rules, we know in the long run we will be wrong only 1 out of 20 times although we will never know which one. This is, of course, only one side of the issue, namely, the consequences of rejecting the null hypothesis on the basis of the 5 percent rule which is the common practice in the medical literature. There is an analogous but not so easily understood error when we accept the null hypothesis. That is, when we think the two samples are drawn from the same population, they may not be.

I believe my point can readily be made by brief quotes from papers written over the past 18 years which have studied the question.

In summary then over a period of more than 30 years the odds are no better than 50-50 that an author's conclusion based on statistical inference was justified. That does not, of course, mean that the conclusion was necessarily wrong. The somewhat lower percentage reported by Gore in 1977 is from the *British Medical Journal.* The British have always paid more attention to teaching statistical methods.

But let us suppose the clinician is lucky and the test result upon which he is relying is indeed correct. How then does he use it in making a decision about his patient? After all, the result from a clinical trial is a group reaction. The study showed that one group fared better than another; that given this treatment, patients, on the average, do better than patients on the average do when given the other therapy. We cannot conclude from that what effect the treatment will have on a particular patient. There is nothing in statistical methodology to provide an answer to that question. But that is precisely the question being asked of the clinician. It is this fact which constitutes the basis of the continuing difference of perspective between the clinician and the statistician. It is essential that the clinician know accurately the probability that the group, to which his patient belongs, will respond to a given intervention.

Table I

Schor, S. and I. Karten. *Journal of the American Medical Association,* March 1966:

Summary of Experience with 10 Journals' Analytic Studies: 149 read—108 not acceptable; 253 errors or 2.34 errors/study—27 percent acceptable.

Schoolman, H. M., et al. *Journal of Laboratory and Clinical Medicine.* March 1968:

Review of the *Journal of Laboratory and Clinical Medicine* indicates an inadequate appreciation of both the purpose and requirements of statistical methods. Current practices have created an extraordinary and indeterminate risk to the reader if he accepts the authors' conclusions. Based on statistical tests of significance, none of the papers reviewed indicate appropriate planning for type II errors.

Gore, S. M., I. G. Jones, and E. C. Rytter. *British Medical Journal.* January 1977.

Sixty-two reports that appeared as papers and originals (excluding short reports) in 13 consecutive issues of the *British Medical Journal* included statistical analysis. Thirty-two had statistical errors of one kind or another; in 18, fairly serious faults were discovered. The summaries of five reports made some claim that was unsupportable on reexamination of the data. Medical investigators should consult with people who have a real understanding of statistical methods throughout their projects. But the problems in interpretation are not limited to type I errors.

Freiman, J. A., T. C. Chalmers, H. Smith, and R. R. Heubler. *New England Journal of Medicine.* September 1978.

Seventy-one "negative" randomized control trails were reexamined to determine if the investigators had studied large enough samples to give a high probability ($>.90$) of detecting a 25 percent and 50 percent therapeutic improvement in response.

Sixty-seven of the trials had a greater than 10 percent risk of missing a true 25 percent therapeutic improvement and with the same risk 50 of the trials could have missed a 50 percent improvement. Thus, many of the therapies labeled as "no different from the control" in trials using inadequate samples have not received a fair test. Concern for the probability of missing an important therapeutic improvement because of small sample sizes deserves more attention in the planning of clinical trials.

Table II
Percent of Papers Studied in Which
Significant Statistical Errors Were Found

Ross, O. B.	*JAMA* 1951	63%
Badgley, R. R.	*Canadian Medical Association Journal* 1961	57%
Schor, S. S.	*JAMA* 1966	52%
Gore, S.	*British Medical Journal* 1977	42%
Giamona	*Clinical Research* 1983	52%

He then knows that on the average, patients of which his patient is one, will respond in a certain way. What this means about his patient is unclear, but some patients of that group will do better and some worse than the average response. The clinician's task is somehow to increase the odds that his particular patient will be one of those who do better.

The clinician has available a great deal more information about his patient than that used to classify the group of which his patient is a member. Moreover, he is continually accumulating new information and can in the context of his knowledge of pathophysiology probe for even more information about this particular patient. The group of which this patient is a member is always grossly defined. The expert clinician subclassifies his patient within the group on the basis of his additional knowledge of the patient. Obviously, it would be wonderful if a controlled clinical trial could be done on this subgroup. Then at least the clinician would know if on the average the subgroup did better than the parent group. But the patient cannot wait—a decision has to be made now. The expert clinician is perceived as expert because of his success in this decision making. In one sense his "expertness" is a reflection of the perception that he does indeed "beat the odds."

At this, the statistician throws up his hands in despair. What can you do with a clinician who wants to countermand a known probability by claiming a subclass probability that cannot be reliably estimated? And how do you guess the error of the clinician's estimate?

The statistician and the clinician have clearly parted company. They are no longer even speaking the same language. The clinician is now not only using a subclass probability that cannot be reliably estimated, he is no longer even talking about probability in the same sense as the statistician, namely relative frequency. Instead, he means by probability a strength of conviction. It is a conviction derived from a hypothesis generated about this particular patient and how well that hypothesis fits an extended set of facts. From this hypothesis the clinician makes a prediction in the form of a tentative diagnosis or an initial therapeutic effort. He continues to add information, some of which he deliberately seeks solely to test the predictions the hypothesis generates.

In the light of these results, he may abandon his original hypothesis and formulate a new one. His management of the patient is thus a series of decisions always mindful of the probabilities of the mean reaction of the large group of which his patient is a member, but always trying to use all the information available to improve the odds of a favorable outcome.

But there remains one more element that must be considered in the decision-making process, namely the importance of the outcome to the patient. This may lead us to decide not for the most probable diagnosis but rather for one for which there is a therapy. In making these sequential decisions which constitute the management of the patient we must, therefore, consider not only the likelihood of any given outcome but its importance. And by importance we mean its importance to the patient not the doctor.

We have thus evolved in this discussion to an informal description of a formal method called decision analysis. In its simplest form, decision analysis states that for a given set of alternatives one need simply multiply the probability of each alternative by the consequences (utility) of that alternative and choose the largest product. Decision analysis has been widely used in industry where the consequences of an outcome (utility) can be quantified as a cost benefit ratio. But how does one quantify the utility in medicine? How do we determine the importance of an outcome to a patient? The easiest and most frequently employed method is for the doctor to consciously or subconsciously make such an estimate. When this is done, there is an invariable and considerable confounding of what is important to the patient with what is important to the doctor. Since the doctor today is almost surely a therapeutic activitist, the resultant utility is much more a reflection of a therapeutic advocate than that of a patient advocate. When one remembers that we are discussing decision making in the face of anxiety provoking uncertainty, it is also clear that part of the utility assessment is a reflection of the doctors dealing with his own anxiety.

But what is the alternative for assessing the patient's utility? Ask the patient? Numerous studies have demonstrated clearly that the person asked would give a different response when healthy than when a patient. Which response should be used? At the moment the best answers are arrived at by, in essence, using both. When the decision would be the same regardless of which was used, the dilemma is resolved. When the decision would be different, the boundaries of the different decision indicate the importance of the difference and afford some guidance as to how to interpret the differences. But research into methods for assigning patient utilities is perhaps the most important aspect of current work in the field.

I have in this brief recitation attempted to trace the scientific base for clinical decision making and to indicate some of its inadequacies. We are confronted with the remarkable situation where this most important of physician functions is neither systematically studied nor taught. Nowhere in the medical curriculum does it explicitly appear. No organizational element exists in the medical school to house those who would pursue these questions, and no career development nor career identification fosters and attracts research and education in clinical decision making. Until these striking deficiencies are corrected, we will continue to rely on an assumed art whose scientific basis is poorly understood not only by medical students but also by their teachers.

26

ETHICAL DILEMMAS OF RESTRICTED RESOURCES

THOMAS C. KING

In 1913, George Bernard Shaw published a prophetic play entitled "The Doctor's Dilemma." Lacing it with a surprising degree of scientific prescience, Shaw presents the dilemma: one dose of curative medicine available; two patients destined to die without it. The patients are opposites in every regard; through their characterizations and the physician's interactions with them, Shaw exposes the human nature of the decisions that physicians must make when needs exceed resources. In a particularly polemic and provocative preface (even for Shaw), he predicts with embarrassing accuracy the evolution the medical profession has undergone since that time. The preface and the play should be required reading for everyone in the business of caring for the sick, particularly for surgeons, a favorite target for Shaw ("The more appalling the mutilation, the more the mutilator is paid!"). In a sometimes perverse way, the work provides a textbook for the physician preparing to face the stream of ethical dilemmas that will confront him in an intensive care unit, particularly when allowances are made for the 80 years that have passed since it was written and for the peculiar political proclivities that guided Shaw at the time (his Fabian socialism and antivivisection causes are especially apparent).

ETHICS AND ADMITTING POLICIES: WHO SHALL LIVE?

How to choose which patient should be admitted to an intensive care unit (ICU) from among the many sick patients who might benefit from those facilities is the modern equivalent of the quandary which formed the focus of Shaw's work. Whenever resources are limited, admission decisions unavoidably involve moral judgments about the value of competing patient's lives and must be made recognizing that in selecting one patient, another is deprived of intensive care. Even in the abstract, it is difficult to establish criteria for admission. Among the criteria to address are the following: What is the likelihood of recovery from the basic disease process? Should patients with "terminal" illness, cancer or cardiac, occupy such facilities even though temporary resuscitation may allow a short-term rehabilitation? And what are "terminal illnesses?" Should any patients with only short-term hope of survival be candidates for admission? What will be the quality of life if survival occurs? How much time will be required in the ICU for successful treatment of the patient's critical illness and how many other patients with shorter-term critical problems might have occupied that bed? How many short-term high-risk, high salvage patients equal one 60-day occupancy? Can a patient's ability to pay for the expensive facilities play any part in the assignment of the ICU bed? With the exceedingly high cost of critical care resources, are those with no or only partial (Medicaid) reimbursement classifications to be necessarily precluded from consideration for such care? With limited resources available and real costs associated with their use, can we be blind to the implications of the payer mix? When priority decisions must be made, can the social "worth" of the patient play any part in deciding who might live?

The immediate assumption in most hospitals is that the sickest patients will be cared for in the ICU; the generalization is rarely workable. There is almost always more demand for beds than there are beds available.

It seems obvious that a competitive admission to the unit should be based on the belief that the specialized care uniquely available in an ICU will have a beneficial effect on the course of the illness and that this effect will be followed by a period of acceptable quality of life after discharge from the unit and the hospital. (Does this require that we categorically deny admission to patients with terminal illnesses?) But when accepting one medically qualified patient means denying another, the ethical judgments involved in the choice may be wrenching.

In establishing priorities for care, even admitting only critically ill patients to the unit may be dangerously inefficient and short-sighted. It may be more logical to admit high-risk patients who are not critically ill as a preventive rather than therapeutic measure. This preventive approach to ICU care may decrease length of stay and preempt the necessity for longer-term admissions if potentially avoidable complications develop. The patient with chronic respiratory disease undergoing an emergency operation may not be in trouble at the close of the case and with attentive and sophisticated care for 48 hours may avoid serious complications. Denied that early intensive care, complications may ensue necessitating prolonged subsequent intensive care and resulting in a higher morbidity and mortality rate. A preventive-admission policy requires that patients who are not critically ill will occasionally get preference over those who are. Can denying the best medical care available in a hospital to a specific, salvageable, critically ill patient in order to maximize the survival rate of the overall population ever be justified?

Ordinarily when man is faced with recurring painful choices, he develops administrative practices to depersonalize the trade-off decisions. Such administrative dodges are common in the management of critical care units. We can escape the ethical judgments surrounding preventive admissions in specific cases by the administrative trick of allocating some beds to such admissions. The ICU director might keep beds filled and announce with regrets to those who request admission for their patients that there are no beds available. Administratively deciding the fate of patients by the accident of first appearance rather than by meritorious judgment may be easier, but is not necessarily preferable.

Reviewing potential admissions against preestablished criteria for patient suitability does not exempt the ICU admitting physician from facing another difficult dilemma: If a bed is empty but the unit is understaffed, should a patient be admitted even if the admission threatens to diminish the adequacy of care being provided to the patients already in the unit? Should an ICU bed be defined as four posts and a mattress? Or must that bed be attached to functioning monitoring equipment and staffed at a nurse-to-patient ratio which allows the high intensity of care appropriate in such units? When monitoring equipment is defective or nursing staff is overworked, should beds be closed in order to maintain the quality of care for the other patients? The admitting physician must make judgments that balance the potential reduction in the adequacy of care for patients already in the unit against the care the denied patient will get in other hospital facilities.

ETHICAL ISSUES IN PATIENT MANAGEMENT

The ethical conflicts are not resolved by the decision to admit a patient. The decision-making process in an ICU is unusual in many ways and results in a variety of special ethical problems. Patients admitted to the ICU usually have altered mental status (because of sedation or the nature of their illness) and consequently cannot share appropriately in decisions about their care. Most are on respirators with endotracheal tubes in place and cannot communicate effectively even when they are alert enough to do so. The rapid action which is sometimes necessary to avert life-threatening complications aggravates this dilemma, as does the fact that many risky invasive procedures are performed often with an urgency which precludes effective involvement of the patient or his family in decisions. The complexity of the problems also often makes it difficult for the patient or family to fully comprehend the issues; this adds to their alienation. This situation places the physician in the position of making decisions of great consequence to the patient without the consultation ordinarily expected in protecting patients' rights.

ETHICAL CONFLICTS IN THE TEAM

Much of the care in intensive care units is administered by critical care specialists and the relationship between the primary physician and the ICU staff is a source of potential conflict. There may be disagreements regarding therapy, timing the discharge of patients from the unit, decisions to reduce the intensity of interventive care, and communication of management decisions to the patient or his family. A new team is now involved, a team which includes not only the primary physician and his or her assistants, but also physicians, nurses, respiratory therapists, and others in the ICU who will assume the major role in the daily care of a patient and become a major source of information for the patient's family. As the size of the team expands, the probability of confusing, conflicting, or inaccurate information being passed on to the patient or his family rises and adds to a family's distress at a time when they are already under severe pressure.

FINANCIAL CONSEQUENCES

Among the most difficult of ethical problems, one for which physicians are particularly ill-trained to deal, has to do with the financial
consequences of the decisions being made. Most patients are now covered by third party payers, but the total cost of intensive care is rarely
covered by that insurance. If the hospitalization is a long one, the
financial burden to the patient or his family may be tremendous. The
fact that a major portion may be covered by insurance and distributed
over a broader population does not vitiate the dilemma, only makes it
less visible. The rapidly escalating insurance premiums over the last
decade must be related in significant degree to the exorbitant costs of
intensive care provided to increasing numbers of patients. Whether
concealed behind the slowly but persistently rising health insurance
rates or felt immediately by the single family unit involved in critical
illness, the physician is making decisions every day that massively increase
costs. Those working in intensive care units who become aware of the
patient and his family's social conditions often discover a man who has
spent his whole life frugally saving for his retirement or to protect his
widow in her old age. He has shared the decisions that led to expenses
for the family unit by careful discussion and analysis with his wife, his
children, his financial advisor, and his attorney. Now, suddenly, decisions of disastrous financial consequences are made by a physician; and
the patient has no chance to share in that decision in any substantial way.
The physician who makes these decisions rarely has any knowledge of
the consequences to the patient or his family of those cost-incurring
decisions. Many families have been financially destroyed by weeks of
costly heroic efforts to resuscitate a dying septuagenarian. Many patients,
when they are coherent and rational, have expressed the desire to limit
heroic efforts in their terminal illness so that they may be saved the
suffering and their family saved the expense of long terminal care. That
a man should have the right to make such decisions seems clear. But
these decisions are rarely communicated to those who make cost-incurring
commitments. The financial security of a lifetime of prudent decision
making is erased by decisions he cannot share in, made by physicians
with no knowledge of the economic consequences of their acts.

The hospital struggling to maintain solvency, is placed in a similar
financially precarious position when the costs are incurred in behalf of
an indigent or uninsured patient. Such patients, victims of street violence,

make up a significant proportion of those trauma patients requiring prolonged intensive care.

RISK–BENEFIT ANALYSIS

Each therapeutic or diagnostic intervention undertaken on a critically ill patient carries the risk that it might complicate the patient's condition, yet it is undertaken with the expectation of benefit. While a major portion of the salvage from an ICU is the direct result of timely and proper selection of dangerous pharmacological or physically invasive procedures, a small but important proportion of the deaths that occur in such units are also the results of those interventions: anticoagulant-induced bleeding, antibiotic-induced renal failure or bone marrow depression, tracheostomy-induced tracheal stenosis or tracheoinnominate artery fistula, and so forth.

Little evidence is available to help us make these risk-benefit decisions on even a meager structure of probability analysis rather than pure intuition. The clinician should weigh the likelihood of survival (and the quality of life should survival occur) against the emotional and financial effects on the patient and the family of the therapy, and he must do so to a distressing degree on the basis of guesses alone.

SUMMARY

The ICU is a microcosm of dilemmas facing the entire medical care system. Among the challenges superficially identified here are pragmatic day-to-day decisions regarding protection of patients' rights, informed consent, conflicts in communication within the medical care team created by extremes of specialization, complications in communicating decisions to patients and their families, mechanisms by which those decisions are made and conflicts adjudicated, the cost-benefit and risk-benefit consequences of decisions, and the ethical agony that requires a physician to make decisions about when to turn off life support systems either to patients directly under his care or (by implication) those he refuses to admit to his jurisdiction. Because there seem to be no solutions to those dilemmas, none are discussed; nor are the fundamental scientific and social questions surrounding how much resource and effort should be expended on the terminal stages of disease in preference to the social and demographic causes of disease. That is the more global analogue of the dilemma Shaw placed before his doctor: If and when society does not have the resources to do everything, what will it do and how will it decide what to do. He correctly predicted we would go on doing things we can do and would rarely ask ourselves whether it was what we ought to do; that we would go on dealing with the little problems that stand up and demand our immediate attention, perhaps as a means of avoiding the larger questions briefly identified here. In the ICU, as in life, we hide from the broader questions while dealing with the immediate questions. We do the best we can with what we see and what we have, and we pay little attention to the ethical consequences, both immediate and long range, of our pragmatic decisions.

27

MEDICAL CARE FOR THE DYING

Eli Ginzberg

What can an economist contribute to a discussion of "Human and Ethical Issues in the Surgical Care of the Patient with Life-Threatening Disease"? The question is especially apposite in the case of an economist who in his long life has never experienced a serious illness and has spent only one night in a hospital. The answer becomes somewhat more obvious when one recalls an earlier presentation that called attention to the changes in the costs of hospital care in the same lifetime.

In the late 1930s a patient with advanced pulmonary disease admitted to the hospital with pneumonia was likely to be dead within 24 hours, and his total bill was between $10 and $20. Today, a patient in the same condition, if placed on a respirator and treated with the full panoply of sophisticated interventions, might be hospitalized for a period of 90 days before death claimed him. The bill in this instance could come to $100,000. Even in an era of annual federal budget deficits of $200 billion, a hospital bill of $100,000 for a single elderly patient with chronic pulmonary disease is a powerful reminder that dollars and health care are inevitably intertwined no matter how much we seek to deny or ignore the linkage.

We know less than we need to know about how the nation's $362 billion of annual health care outlays (1983) are distributed among different categories of patients—the well, the indisposed, the seriously ill and the moribund. But some simple arithmetic examples can be illuminating and we do have a few figures that shed indirect light on patients with life-threatening diseases.

177

An expenditure of $362 billion for a population of approximately 235 million means that on average health care outlays amount to over $1500 per person, $6000 per family of four.[1] That, however, is a national average. Take New York City: I have recently calculated that total health care outlays in New York approximated $17 billion in 1983. With a resident population of 7 million the cost comes to just under $10,000 per family of four. Since hospitals in New York City also provide considerable care for nonresidents, a more valid figure might be between $8500 and $9000 per resident family of four.

The distinguished health economist, Victor Fuchs of Stanford University, has recently called attention to the fact that our presumption that the elderly are heavy consumers of health care may be a misinterpretation of the data that indicate that 30 percent of all health care services are furnished to people over 65 who account for about 11 percent of the population.[2] Fuchs does not challenge the figures but rather the inference. He suggests that the high users of health care are not the elderly per se, but rather individuals who are in the last year or two of their lives. Since most people who die are elderly, we have confused large outlays in the final months before death with high medical expenditures of the elderly.

There are several pieces of data that support Fuchs' hypothesis. The first points to the fact that 6 percent of all aged Medicare enrollees (i.e., excluding the disabled) account for over 50 percent of all Medicare expenditures.[3] Another relates to the difference between expenditures for hospitalized Medicare patients who survive versus those who die in the course of the year. The latter have total reimburseable expenditures six to seven times those of the former.[4]

Still another finding: An earlier study revealed that one in four Medicare enrollees who died within the course of the study year had high reimbursable expenses ($5000 or more).[5] For those who survived the year the ratio was only 1 in 25. In short, nonsurvivors are over six times more prominent among the high-cost patient group. And among the nonsurvivors, half of all their costs are incurred during the two months immediately preceding death.

The findings, even though stitched together from different cross-sectional studies and undertaken over a period of years during which the value of the dollar declined and the costs of medical care increased, cumulatively speak to the high costs incurred by patients during their final year of life, in particular their last 60 days.

Classifying patients as moribund and estimating their medical expenditures during the last year or last two months of life can only be done retrospectively. The patient who is seriously ill and who succumbs after 60 days or so can be defined as having been moribund in the period immediately preceding death. But clearly the term moribund cannot be applied to the seriously ill patient who is treated, leaves the hospital, and makes even a partial recovery.

We are frequently reminded that our British cousins, faced with a severe stringency in resources for their health care system, have no option but to adopt a rationing approach when it comes to treating the elderly.[6] They use chronological age to determine whether costly treatment modalities such as renal dialysis, open-heart surgery, organ transplants, hip replacements should or should not be undertaken. We have not had to confront the rationing issue up to this point other than for exceptional procedures such as heart transplants. What the future may bring, however, is far from certain because potential treatments may be limited as much or more by a shortage of organs as by a shortage of dollars.

The question that should be raised is whether it makes sense from the vantage of the individual and the society that every patient have the benefit of the full panoply of sophisticated medical care irrespective of age, physical condition, and prospects of gaining or regaining functionality. Let us consider briefly the following cases.

The recent conflicts over "Baby Doe" cases leave little question that a significant portion of the citizenry believes that parents should be permitted to refuse life-sustaining treatment for severely impaired infants who have little or no promise of ever being able to function effectively. Admittedly, another part of the citizenry has a different view. The question that our society must face, sooner rather than later, is whether the prolongation of life, or a minimum quality of life, should be the goal of medical intervention.

Consider the opposite end of the spectrum, the case of a ninety-year-old woman operated for cancer in her forties, who has enjoyed a symptom-free existence until the recent emergence of a new tumor. Her physician believes that an operation may relieve her pain and extend her life. However, if surgery is ventured, it may be found that the cancer is not excisable. An alternative course would be to control her pain with narcotics.

I suggest that the decision in this case should rest, in the first instance, with the patient. Moreover, it would not be unreasonable if in reaching a decision she considered the economic implications of the alternatives. If the surgery and the after-care threatened to make serious inroads into her modest savings, she might decide against surgery with an aim of assuring that her funds be used to pay for the college expenses of a grandchild. Many people in their nineties, even those who are seriously ill, are prepared for death, at least they see little point in struggling to delay it.

The medical journals, the press, and even the courts are becoming increasingly entangled in questions of choice and decision-making affecting the treatment or nontreatment of seriously ill and moribund patients. It would be unrealistic to search for a single criterion, such as maximum treatment aimed at prolonging life or freedom of choice for the individual (or his surrogate) to terminate treatment. In the face of ever more sophisticated technology that can prolong life but that often cannot contribute to the restoration of functionality, different individuals will feel differently about further medical intervention. Considerations of money aside, these differences in values are, and will long remain, sources of conflict that require continuing reassessment and resolution.

A few concluding observations. In previous generations there was relatively little that the physician could do to prolong the life of the dying patient. But to the extent that he had some scope for judgment and action, he did not hesitate to do what he believed his patient and the family desired. In an era in which many patients no longer have a family physician who knows them well, the physician is less inclined to assume such responsibility, the more so in the presence of widespread malpractice suits.

One must also take note of the fact that in recent decades, more and more patients die in a hospital, a great many in teaching hospitals where residents have considerable influence on the course of treatment. Residents are at a stage in their careers when the potential rather than the limitations of medicine dominates their judgment. Hence, they are inclined to do more and more even when an older and wiser physician would be inclined to favor the termination of treatment. We may be at the point where a moribund patient who wishes to die without harassment and with dignity must remain at home or spend his last days in a hospice where bold medical maneuvers are impractical and/or countermanded.

Finally, we will probably gain a better understanding of how to face death now that more and more of the population is living into their seventies and eighties, even into their nineties. In the last century, death took a great many infants and children and many adults in the middle years. We accepted the first and sought to deny the second. We are only now approaching the point where most people will die after having reached three-score and ten and the favored, four-score. We have a lot still to learn about how to deal with death among the elderly.

NOTES

1. Projected figure. Mark Freeland and Carol Ellen Schendler, "National Health Expenditure Growth in the 1980s: An Aging Population, New Technologies, and Increasing Competition," *Health Care Financing Review,* March 1983.
2. Victor R. Fuchs, "A Note on Age, Survival Status and Health Care Expenditures," September 13, 1983 (unpublished).
3. "The Medicare and Medicaid Data Book, 1983," *Health Care Financing Program Statistics,* December 1983.
4. Jim Lubitz and Ronald Prihoda, "Use and Costs of Medicare Services in the Last 2 Years of Life," *Health Care Financing Review,* Spring 1984.
5. Charles Helbing, "Medicare: Use and Reimbursement for Aged Persons by Survival Status, 1979," *Health Care Financing Notes,* November 1983.
6. Henry J. Aaron and William B. Schwartz, *The Painful Prescription: Rationing Hospital Care* (Washington, D.C.: Brookings Institution, 1984).

28

EXPERIMENTAL SURGERY: WHAT IS IT?

KEITH REEMTSMA

What is experimental surgery? An appendectomy for acute appendicitis is *not* experimental surgery. Implanting an artificial heart in a human patient *is* experimental surgery. But there is a vast in-between area.

As defined in the Nuremburg Code and in the Helsinki Declaration following World War II, experimental medicine was divided into two general areas. The first involved experiments done for the sake of information but without benefit to the patient. The second involved the use of procedures of unproven value that are performed for the benefit of the patient. But what should constitute "proof"?

This is not easy to define. Some would require randomized, prospective trials for proof. In the case of treatment of bleeding esophageal varices, it is now generally believed on the basis of randomized trials that it does not make much difference what procedure is done. The outcome is determined by the extent of liver disease. Another example would be the use of randomization of surgical procedures performed in the treatment of breast cancer. However, there are other circumstances in which randomization is inappropriate. I shall cite several examples.

A 14-year-old child with aortic stenosis requires surgery. There are two ways to approach her problem, either to replace the valve or to open the valve. The decision must be made at the operating table. It would be unacceptable to randomize patients such as this before the operation. The decision has to be made on the basis of the findings at the operating table.

183

A young man in his thirties had been in our Coronary Care Unit for three weeks and on heavy doses of vasopressors during the last week. An appropriate donor heart was found and was transplanted into him. It seems to me that there are conditions such as end-stage cardiac disease in which the outcome is so well-known that it would be unethical to deny the patient a heart transplant because it had been decided that the patient would be placed into a randomized prospective study. My plea is that we use common sense in our search for proof.

I believe in the statistical approach to certain scientific problems, and it is particularly applicable in the use of various medications and vaccines. Randomization is much less practical in many of the conditions that surgeons deal with, such as end-stage organ failure. In such cases, it would be inappropriate to deny the importance and validity of pilot studies, particularly when the endpoint without the operation is well known.

We know that patients who are entered into cardiac transplantation studies and do not receive a heart transplant have a 90 percent mortality rate within three months. If they receive the heart transplant, they have a one-year survival rate of 80–90 percent. This experience emphasizes the point that procedures that may be classified as experimental can have excellent outcomes; conversely, certain procedures that are considered standard may have unsatisfactory survival figures. Examples are surgical procedures for carcinoma of the esophogus and pancreas.

My plea would be that we do not become too rigid. The major risk faced by patients is not from unrandomized or unregulated studies. Peer review and malpractice suits are excellent safeguards against overly venturesome surgeons. The greater danger today is from overregulation. I would hope that we do not see overregulation affect the development of procedures as it has the development of pharmaceuticals in the United States.

Part VII
EDUCATION IN THANATOLOGY:
LEARNING TO COPE WITH DEATH,
DYING, AND BEREAVEMENT

29

COMPREHENSION OF DEATH AND BEREAVEMENT

Vanderlyn R. Pine

Comprehending death is a complex multidimensional process. Even so, at the everyday level most of us have to grapple with the process frequently and often painfully. We are exposed to death when we read the newspapers, watch television, listen to the radio, hear of dying friends or acquaintances, visit people in hospitals, go to funerals, drive past cemeteries, see dead animals, and so forth. All such awarenesses are part of this complex psychosocial process. Furthermore, most of us use believable organizing frameworks, hypothetical models, or plausible explanatory theories to help cope with and understand death and bereavement.

The purpose of this chapter is to explore and discuss some of the everyday, often taken-for-granted aspects of life and consciousness that have an impact on our comprehension of death, bereavement, and grief. Inherent in this objective is the need to demonstrate (1) the importance of understanding the reasoning processes surrounding death and (2) the intricate connection between these processes and our attempts to "explain" death to ourselves and others. In the same vein, distinctions between intellectual, social, and emotional understanding are presented to assist in the clarification of death comprehension. To accomplish this, an overview of the hypotheses, theories, and empirical findings of some well-known death scholars is presented. Drawing from these writings and the outcomes of many death and bereavement studies, a suggested protocol is offered for professionals dealing with both dying and bereaved people.

DEATH AND THE REASONING PROCESS

There are at least three models of the reasoning process that can be used to help understand death. First, there is the deductive reasoning model, which occurs when one possesses a general concept or understanding of death and then particularizes it for a given person's death. For example, employing the reasoning that everyone must die some day may help us understand that the death of a specific person is a natural consequence of life. Second, there is the inductive reasoning model which occurs when one infers something from a specific person's death and then generalizes that everyone must die. For example, when we know that a particular person has died, eventually we may come to understand that death will happen to all of us. Third, there is the retroductive reasoning model which occurs when we look at a death event and then seek to find logical reasons for its occurrence. For example, when we know that a loved person has died, we may "look back" to try to understand the plausible reasons for the death having occurred.

The point of considering the reasoning process and our understanding of death is neither philosophical nor esoteric, although the actual process is both. Quite simply, it is important because death is brought into our consciousness through a combination of the three reasoning styles. Other ideas about death may emerge from our belief in widespread, culturally accepted theories about God or the universe, and then we deduce ideas about specific deaths (deduction). From a specific individual's death we gain understanding that all of us will die some day (induction). We gain additional understanding through the process of trying to "figure out and explain to ourselves" a death, and this act of putting a death into our own common sense perspective may help us come to grips with death (retroduction). The real life process of comprehending death actually involves a complex mixture of all three reasoning models.

Basic premises we make about the nature of humankind also influence and help us form our theories of death. For example, acceptance of the premise that death is inevitable generally facilitates a more realistic attitude toward one's own death. A belief in immortality leads to an additional perception of death. Recently, however, many of our premises and hypotheses concerning death have become inappropriate and obsolete. High technology, prolongevity, and artificial life have rendered our past views of death outdated. Today, many people feel that death is appropriate only at a certain time in life and only for certain people. For instance, some may feel that death is "appropriate" for a ninety year old whereas the death of a teenager is viewed by many as unexpected and inappropriate.

Our theories about bereavement and grief also influence how we react to and comprehend death situations. To help make life more meaningful and to assist in understanding death requires that we evaluate our theories about death, grief, and bereavement. Moreover, it is important, especially for professionals, to examine their own theories about death in order to deal with death issues more adequately. This is the case because all of us, including professional care providers, someday must cope with death on the everyday, pragmatic level.

EXPLANATORY THEORIES ABOUT DEATH

An explanatory theory helps us comprehend death and bereavement. Such a theory is used by people individually, institutionally, and societally to aid in the grief process. For our purposes, explanation involves examining many different aspects of a situation or event simultaneously and then trying to make sense out of them. Explanatory theories also involve examining all the *relationships* among the different aspects of the death event. Put simply, explanatory theories seek to answer such questions as "why" concerning death, "how" to handle bereavement and grief, and so forth.

There are many different explanatory theories of death, but for this discussion, we will mention the six most common ones. Each or a combination of several may be utilized to help comprehend death. People in everyday situations use such theories in a common sense attempt to cope with death events that they experience.[1]

Religious explanations that view the power of a higher being or God as causal can be used. The intent of these explanations is to provide a means of assuaging grief, e.g., "It was God's will that she died, and God will help you through your grief."

Medical explanations that view death as a result of pathology (illness) and grief as an illness which can be "cured" medically can be used. The latter often leads to the practice of medicating the bereaved and this may facilitate forgetting and/or escaping from the grief temporarily.

Ethological explanations that approach the death and grief issues as instinctive and characteristic of the human race also may be utilized.

Psychological explanations are used by some people and seek to illustrate that death and grief are emotive and cognitive responses.

Sociological explanations that perceive death as a social event and process can be used. From this perspective, mourning and grief are viewed as social behavior in response to death.

Psychosocial explanations that view death as a trigger or stimulus and grief as an emotional response in a particular societal cultural setting can be used as well.[2]

Of course, it is possible (perhaps even common) to use more than one of the above explanations simultaneously. This is especially true when death touches on the multiple dimensions of one's life, which in "reality" is usually the case. Furthermore, the basis of comprehension is a compilation of all dimensions and elements in a person's life.

COMPREHENDING DEATH

Comprehension is the act of recognizing and processing the nature and significance of a concept, in this case, death. The dynamics of attaining personal and interpersonal meanings of death and bereavement are intricate, complicated, and often emotionally and physically draining. Thus, as we pass through life events, we use past experiences, organizing models, our emotional reactions, and a vast repertoire of personal responses as a foundation from which our psychosocial reactions evolve. The significance of each previous event then becomes a component in future situations in which we must "comprehend" similar events.

When referring to comprehension, there is a tendency to think only in terms of an intellectual understanding. However, reliance on this intellectual perspective as the sole means of understanding can bring about at least three interrelated problems which can have a negative impact on one's outlook on death. First, there may be the fallacy of "misplaced concreteness." This occurs when an individual believes that his or her own theory about death is the only answer. By treating any explanatory theory as if it were etched in concrete weakens one's ability to adjust to death.

Second, there may be the error of believing in "the right way." This happens when one feels there is only one route to follow in comprehending death to the exclusion of any other options or alternatives. Generally, this does not take place for malevolent reasons but rather because a person may feel duty-bound to accomplish a specific goal by a prescribed singular method.

Third, there may be a "failure to recognize individuality." The uniqueness and specific needs of each individual must be taken into consideration in order to deal with death in a healthy fashion. Hence, each person's reactions to a particular death may differ considerably from all others to the same death.

Another necessary aspect of comprehension is an understanding of the powerful emotions involved in bereavement. For example, rather than simply acknowledging the need to cry, it is crucial to address the complex and multidimensional cognitive elements of death awareness as well. As professional care providers, it is not enough just to enable a bereaved person to cry; the bereaved should be helped to attain a cognitive understanding of why they are crying and to determine the personal meaning of their crying. In other words, while an initial emotive step may be crying, the next step is knowing the significance of the crying.

Furthermore, "just crying" may not be sufficient for the expression of one's emotions, and the additional release of feelings may be warranted. Other forms of release can include screaming, striking at something, writing out one's feelings about the loss, and so forth.

In addition, there is the problem of oversimplification of the concepts of bereavement and grief. This refers to the acceptance and blind application of models using *rigid* steps, stages, and sequences to "explain away" grief. Grief models and theories can be utilized in an appropriate manner, but there are some dangers of which we should be aware. These models need not be adhered to precisely but should serve as working hypotheses. It also should be noted that when a care provider selects a specific model, and it does not work, it should be discarded and a different model or approach should be considered for use.

The most hopeful aspect of these points is that new, worthwhile models of death comprehension will emerge if they are acknowledged and encouraged. Clearly, this places the onus of responsibility on professionals who study and write about death as well as those who are care providers.

STUDYING GRIEF

To help understand death, bereavement, and grief more fully, it is helpful to review the salient points that some of the most important theorists and practitioners have observed. In this section, let us turn our attention to the writings of a small but significant number of noted death scholars. Their works can be integrated in a constellation of theories which helps us explain and comprehend death.

Let us begin with the writings of Emile Durkheim, who analyzed funeral rites and mourning behavior in *The Elementary Forms of Religious Life*. He points out that funeral rites are ceremonies which designate a state of "uneasiness or sadness" (1915:435). The implication is that death produces personal anxieties which are addressed by the funeral ceremony, which in turn, is indicative of a society's feelings about and comprehension of death. Through a comparative study of funeral rituals, Durkheim illustrates that these rites mirror a particular society's concepts about and interpretation of life and death.

According to Durkheim, mourning behavior is neither a natural reaction nor a spontaneous release of emotions. He argues that the bereaved are actors who feel obliged to "play out" their emotions through gestures that are sanctioned by society. In other words, if a bereaved person does not display his or her grief in an acceptable manner the community will show its disapproval or impose some sort of punishment. Hence, Durkheim posits:

> Mourning is not a natural movement of private feelings wounded by a cruel loss; it is a duty imposed by the group. One weeps, not simply because he is sad, but because he is forced to weep. It is a ritual attitude which he is forced to adopt out of respect for custom, but which is, in a large measure, independent of his affective state (p. 443).

Sigmund Freud analyzes grief in "Mourning and Melancholia" (1959). He identifies grief as a "painful" state of mind and refers to grief in terms of the "economics of the mind" (1959:153). Using the concept of economics allows Freud to treat grief as part of a psychological exchange process with tasks and activities being carried out as "labour" in exchange for a kind of psychic "freedom" from the dead person.

The goal of what Freud (p. 156–161) referred to as "the work of grief" is to free the bereaved person from the attachments to the dead person, the inhibitions of becoming a separate being, and conflicts of ambivalence over the lost love relationship. Therefore, "the work of mourning" is a temporal process occurring over time. According to Freud's theory (p. 163), after "normal grief" accomplishes the "labour" of freeing the bereaved from the dead person, it does not leave "traces of any gross change" in the bereaved person. This has led some to interpret that completed grief work represents a cured condition. I do not believe that Freud intended for this interpretation to be used by clinicians who view grief as "curable" in the medical sense implying that it is an "illness." He posited that the human psyche has the *ability to cope naturally* with loss.

Freud recognized that it is not beneficial to try to utilize a chronological time limit to describe the duration of "normal" grief. Expanding upon Freud helps clarify our position regarding the difficulty of measuring psychosocial time in contrast to the easily measurable chronological time. Freud's view is that completing the *process* of grief work determines the time limit of the duration of "normal grief." Hence, when the process has occurred, then enough time will have passed in which to complete the three essential tasks of grief work—freedom, separation, and coping with ambivalence.[3]

Bronislaw Malinowski notes the strong impact on and the ways in which *society* is affected by death in *Magic, Science, and Religion*. He observes:

> (Death)... threatens the very cohesion and solidarity of the group... (and the funeral) counteracts the centrifugal forces of fear, demoralization, and provides the most powerful means of reintegration of the group's shaken solidarity and of reestablishment (1948:53).

Malinowski (p. 52) goes on to state that the despair, the funeral ceremonies, and the mourning behavior all serve to demonstrate the emotions of the bereaved and the loss experienced by the whole group. These aspects of death reinforce as well as reflect the natural feelings of the survivors. The death rites create a social event out of a natural act, for it is only natural to die.[4]

In most societies, it is during the funeral ceremony that death reactions become visible. Funeral rites provide bereaved people with a defined social role that functions to help them pass through a period of adjustment following the death. The rites also delimit the period of mourning, allow the bereaved to release their grief emotions publicly, and aim at helping to commemorate an individual's death.[5]

Erich Lindemann's analysis of the symptoms and handling of grief entitled "The Symptomatology and Management of Acute Grief," is theoretically sound, empirically grounded, and clearly written. Lindemann (1944) discusses many aspects of grief, but, more importantly, he distinguishes between normal and pathological grief. He delineates ways of dealing with repressed and delayed grief, both of which are common problems, and observes that grief can precede a loss, a condition he calls "anticipatory grief." In addition, Lindemann emphasizes that grief may be an *acute* psychosocial condition. The realities of modern war and mass societal trauma are precursors of acute grief which is characterized by a rapid onset, serious conditions, and treatable symptoms.

Lindemann explains that acute grief is an observable syndrome with psychological and somatic symptoms that may appear immediately, may be delayed, exaggerated, or apparently absent. Furthermore, distorted reactions may occur and can be viewed as a specific aspect of the grief syndrome. Lindemann believes that with appropriate psychiatric intervention distorted grief may be transformed into normal grief with the possibility of resolution. In other words, Lindemann feels that with comprehension, understanding, *and* clinical intervention, unresolved grief is manageable.

Lindemann (p. 143) goes on to point out that the duration of grief reactions depends on how well the bereaved person performs "grief work." The resolution of grief may be subverted when bereaved people try to avoid carrying out grief work because of the distress and emotional energy required to complete it.

By resolution Lindemann (p. 143) means achieving "emancipation from the *bondage* to the deceased," readjustment to the environment, and the ability to form new relationships. The idea that the dead person holds the bereaved "in bondage" refers to the interpersonal relationship between people. In this sense, bondage emerges from power so dominant that the dead person remains not only in the bereaved person's memory but also in control of the bereaved person's life.

According to Lindemann, it is possible to predict the type and severity of a distorted grief reaction from information and knowledge about the premorbid personality of the bereaved. For example, the extent of the affective (love/hate) relationship to the deceased is an important factor in determining the severity of the grief reaction. Also, he found that patients with obsessive or depressive personalities often experience agitated depression after bereavement.

One of Lindemann's major contributions to grief studies involves the concept of management. He explains that with proper management severe psychosomatic and/or medical problems stemming from distorted grief can be avoided, ameliorated, or eliminated. Among other things, the psychiatrist, psychologist, or other professional can help "share" the grief work by helping the bereaved person extricate him or herself from over-attachment to the dead person. Lindemann (p. 147) states that the bereaved need to accept the pain of their loss, review their (past) relationship with the deceased, and realize that there will be changes in their expressions of emotional reactions. The bereaved need to "talk through" their sense of loss and sorrow. Moreover, the professional care provider should encourage new patterns of conduct for the bereaved in their new life without the deceased person.[6]

Raymond Firth observes that not only psychological elements are essential for the benefit of the living. He emphasizes that there are societal elements that help resolve many of their ambivalent feelings about death. Firth notes in *Elements of Social Organization:*

> A funeral ritual is a social rite par excellence. Its ostensible object is the dead person, but it benefits not the dead, but the living ... it is those who are left behind—the kinsfolk, the neighbors, and other members of the community— for whom the ceremony is really performed (1964:63).

Firth (p. 63) continues to state that the funeral supplies three necessary elements to the living. The first element is the resolution of uncertainties in the behavior of the immediate kin. The funeral provides relatives with an opportunity to publicly display their grief and sets a period of time on their (public) mourning. As such, it is a ritual of closure.

Firth refers to the second element as the fulfillment of social consequence, which means that the ceremony helps to reinforce the appropriate attitudes of the members of society to each other. Although stressing the dead, the funeral points out the value of the services of the living.

The third element is the economic aspect. Every funeral involves the expenditure of money, goods, and services. Analytically, this ties in with Freud's reference to the concept of economics and the exchange process in relation to grief and mourning. Freud notes that the bereaved feel they must "compensate" in some way for the death. He was referring to the psychological exchange process. Firth, on the other hand, states that the exchange process is important to the bereaved on a tangible social and economic level as well. Bereaved people may feel the need to make restitution to the deceased by purchasing such nonabstract items as funeral feasts, funeral merchandise, religious services, and so forth.

John Bowlby's analysis of the nature of human attachment entitled, *Attachment* (1969), draws on numerous studies about separation and loss in early childhood. He delineates patterns that occur regularly in early childhood and then traces how similar patterns of response can be observed later in the functioning of the adult personality. He begins not with a symptom or syndrome, but with an experience he believes to have pathogenic potential for the emerging personality, that is, the loss of a mother figure when a child is between six months and six years of age.

Bowlby reasons (p. 350) that attachment behavior persists throughout childhood and also throughout life, for "old and new figures are selected and proximity and communication maintained with them." The result-ant behavior remains the same but the means for achieving it become diversified as the maturing child incorporates new elements of attach-ment behavior. Bowlby links ongoing and new attachments to the experi-ence of loss. Moreover, he demonstrates that without attachment, there cannot be loss. Using Bowlby's framework, the absence of continuing physical proximity and the lack of communication defines the meaning of loss.

Colin Murray Parkes' analysis entitled *Bereavement: Studies of Grief in Adult Life* (1972) gives an excellent review of the literature on the psychol-ogy of grief. Not only is Bowlby's influence evident; it also is acknowl-edged by Parkes. His major focus is on the loss of a spouse. Parkes' position is that grief is a functional disorder, is of specific etiology, has recognizable features, and has a fairly predictable course. He emphasizes the paradox that even with these characteristics, grief is neglected in the psychiatric literature.

Parkes presents two additional elements that he feels influence the reaction to bereavement. One of these elements he calls "stigma," and it is reflective of the social attitude of ostracism in the treatment of the newly bereaved person. People often avoid the bereaved person or feel uncomfortable in his or her presence. The not-so-hidden meaning is that the bereaved person is viewed by others as tainted in some awful way by the death of a loved one.

Parkes calls the other element "deprivation," and this refers to the absence of those psychosocial supplies such as love and security that were provided by the dead person. By identifying the deprivation factor, Parkes provides a critical link between grief and bereavement. Bereave-ment is equivalent to deprivation in the objective sense because it repre-sents a measurable or actual loss. Grief, on the other hand, is a psychosocial response to loss. This distinction helps clinicians recognize the observable elements of a particular bereavement and its losses and then to treat the attendant psychosocial grief reactions.

Parkes considers defense mechanisms of the newly bereaved such as disbelief and selective forgetting, to be coping strategies that the bereaved use to alleviate the pain of grief. Furthermore, he does not consider them to be "pathological." He states that some losses are never totally "gotten over" and that this is not necessarily abnormal or pathological. Instead, there is a consciousness that a loss has occurred and that it is part of the reality of life. Therefore, "acceptance" of a loss does not require "getting over it" but rather coping with the loss so that daily life can go on.

Parkes notes that the effects of ambivalence, the inability to communicate, and the absence of understood social expectations and acceptable rituals for mourning are likely to foster pathological reactions to bereavement. He feels that therapists dealing with grief reactions should assume an accepting attitude in order to enable the bereaved person to feel free to express feelings of anger, guilt, despair, and anxiety. This should promote the transformation of pathological grief into normal grief, and then the bereaved can be directed toward resolution.

There are many other treatments of grief and bereavement which could be examined; however, the major points raised thus far cover the essential factors that aid in our goal of explicating comprehension of death, bereavement, and grief.

THE OUTCOMES OF GRIEF STUDIES

Many of the theoretical and practical perspectives can be integrated and extended into a coherent framework through which we can gain a fuller comprehension of death and grief. The following hypotheses are drawn from an interpretive coalescence of the works already cited plus personal observation and theorizing on the critical issues noted in them. Two of the serious drawbacks of much of the present-day literature involve the unlinked use of theory and evidence. On the one hand, using pure theory about death may make good philosophy but may fall short of being helpful at the everyday level. On the other hand, using only empirical evidence or experience may be temporarily helpful but may miss many of the important complexities involved. Our goal, therefore, is to bridge gaps between the strictly theoretical and the strictly empirical by offering an integrated constellation of usable hypotheses to help in our understanding and comprehension of death.

All the evidence indicates that grief can be resolved. Not surprisingly, there is a definitional problem with the term "resolution." It does *not* mean that a bereaved person will actually "get over" the pain of grief and will never experience pain again in connection with the death. Rather, it means that a bereaved person reaches a point at which the pain of a particular death can be accepted and can be "lived with." When this occurs, the bereaved person comprehends that life can continue, although in an altered state, without the one who has died.

Most perspectives agree that death and grief should be shared openly with other people. One problematic aspect of this issue is timing. For instance, a problem may occur when different members of a family experience different grief reactions at different points in time. Although such reactions may not be shared easily, it is beneficial when they are mutually comprehended, understood, and accepted. The matter of psychosocial timing is of great importance to both care providers and the people experiencing and attempting to share these reactions.

Another dimension connected with the issue of shared grief is the communication process itself. Open communication allows for and promotes expressions of differences in style, intensity, and depth of grief. Open communication is the most sensible avenue to follow in attempting to recognize and cope with these and other differences in people.

Most writings confirm that anticipatory responses to a potential death should be recognized as a form of actual grief. The so-called anticipatory grief process should be considered a beneficial and necessary step toward resolution. Although anticipatory grief generally can be a positive experience there are two potential problems. One, *too much* anticipatory grief response may be detrimental. Excessive anticipation can result in family and friends emotionally and physically distancing themselves from the dying person "too soon," causing the dying person to feel abandoned and isolated. Two, when very intense anticipatory grief occurs, other members of the dying person's family or social milieu may feel ignored and unimportant. Unfortunately, there is no guideline to determine the correct amount of anticipatory grief that is beneficial.

The evidence suggests that children should be included in death-related grief work, regardless of their age. When dealing with children who are experiencing grief, adults should strive to confront issues that elicit their own feelings of anxiety and discomfort. Adults should respond to all questions with honesty and directness. In this regard, it is advisable to use "gentle honesty" in response to inquiries from young children. Gentle honesty refers to responding truthfully to a child's question "just a little bit at a time." This calls for listening to the child to determine what and how much information he or she wants. Many questions about death do not call for long, detailed, or in-depth answers, and such a response is neither necessary nor expected by the child.

The evidence indicates that professional intervention can be helpful in the death-related grief process and should be initiated when it is warranted. Assistance can be given by many different care-providing occupations including physicians, nurses, clergy, social workers, funeral directors, hospice workers, family therapists, and grief counselors. Conversely, it should be recognized that these providers of counseling and assistance are not impervious to the pain of grief and that professionals may need help in dealing with their own grief.

There are self-help groups to help the dead person's family help cope with death, as well as self-help groups to assist care providers in dealing with the deaths of their patients or clients. The self-help groups that deal with death concerns include organizations such as The Compassionate Friends, Widow-To-Widow, SIDS Support Groups, Candlelighters, volunteer hospice groups, and others. These organizations offer interactive membership with participatory activities and peer counseling.[7]

This constellation provides us with a loosely organized body of knowledge with a reasonable theoretical base and an emerging empirical orientation. It also gives rise to an inevitable question—How can professionals benefit from utilizing the preceding theories about comprehension of death to deal with grief?

SUGGESTED PROTOCOL FOR PROFESSIONALS

Based on a wide range of theoretical and clinical studies, research experience, and personal observations, the following suggested protocol for professionals dealing with the bereaved is offered.[8]

1. Death education and training are necessary. Ignorance of the grief process on the part of professionals can be counterproductive and potentially harmful to the bereaved. Hence, a coherent program of professional education is a worthwhile endeavor. Today, more than forty years after Lindemann's seminal writings, only a meager percentage of medical schools offer an entire course on death and dying to their students.

2. The immediacy issue in respect to intervention is of critical importance. Specifically, it is best to intervene as soon as possible after the loss, when professional assistance is needed. The rationale behind this is simple. Rather than let problems compound, multiply, and snowball until the resolution of problematic grief reactions may seem impossible, it is advisable to intervene as soon as it is detected that professional care would be beneficial.

3. Health care professionals should form interdisciplinary approaches to care for the dying and the bereaved. Specifically, this means there should be an effort to provide integrated sources of emotional support. This effort requires directed leadership from the highest levels of health care administration. It also requires interdisciplinary commitment to common problem-solving issues such as levels of patient care, coordinated services, professional burnout, and so forth.

4. Professionals should provide consistent emotional support to family and important others before (when possible) and after the death rather than at the time of a later emotional crisis or at sporadic intervals.

5. Professional intervention techniques should assess and take into consideration the home situation and social environment of the family.

6. Formal follow-up procedures for grief counseling should be established and provided to the bereaved. For example, in addition to immediate death needs, services such as anniversary counseling also should be provided.

7. The communication process is a critical part of the mourning experience. This means that openness, honesty, and directness are of great importance. One must be careful neither to trivialize the death nor to overstate its tragic consequences.

8. All relevant conditions, symptoms, and anticipated reactions of both the dying person and the bereaved survivors should be explained to and understood by all parties.

CONCLUDING COMMENTS

The matter of death comprehension is complex, multifaceted, and involves numerous psychological, social, and cultural dimensions. It has been suggested in this chapter that through a combination of inductive, deductive, and retroductive reasoning people utilize their basic premises about life in general and death in particular to help form a personal understanding of death. Furthermore, it is argued that people develop various methods of coping with life and death events in accordance with the compatibility of these reasoning approaches with their beliefs, values, and sociocultural backgrounds. Hence, there is widespread usage of everyday theories which focus on major explanatory themes such as theology, medicine, ethology, psychology, sociology, and social psychology.

Comprehending death requires at least three levels of understanding, each important in its own right as well as in conjunction with the others. Out of this perspective comes the belief that people need to develop the skills to foster personal cognition or comprehension of death and bereavement that is intellectually grounded, socially and culturally based, and psychologically appropriate for themselves.

The ideas and observations of great thinkers are useful as a springboard for further advancement in the field of death and bereavement. Beyond that, it is the essential clarity, logic, and believability of their writings that make their ideas so beneficial in establishing the present integrated perspective. Their works blend together in a mosaic of themes woven into a pattern of coping strategies for dying, death, bereavement, and grief. Hopefully, some new ideas will be generated from the grief studies discussed in this chapter.

Finally, although it is risky business to give general advice on a subject so complex but at the same time so individual as death, a protocol for professionals has been offered. It seems worth taking the risk if it can be helpful in facilitating the difficult transitions caused by death and bereavement.

NOTES

1. Although the publication did not come to my attention until the present position was developed, for an alternative discussion of "Explanatory Models of the Bereavement Process" see the recent treatment of this subject in Osterweis, Solomon, & Green (eds.), *Bereavement: Reactions, Consequences, and Care,* (Washington, D.C.: National Academy Press, 1984), pp. 56–58.
2. These brief descriptions are simplified versions which have not been fully developed in this chapter. However, their utility and applicability in an everyday context can be identified easily.
3. Buttressing my perspective on independently developed grounds, this point is similarly recognized in Osterweis, Solomon, & Green (eds.), *Bereavement: Reactions, Consequences, and Care, op. cit.,* pp. 52–53.
4. Both Durkheim and Malinowski were concerned with that which could be considered "natural." Malinowski referred to death and its attendant ceremonies as

"natural" events whereas Durkheim argued that mourning should not be considered "natural" in the instinctive sense but, rather as learned behavior. It is not necessary for us to reconcile their views, since both perspectives can fit into this article's overall framework.

5. This issue is much broader than presently discussed. For a more complete treatment see Vanderlyn R. Pine, "Social Organization and Death," in *Omega*, 1972, Vol. 3, No. 2, pp. 150–151. For a much-expanded treatment which integrates psychological and sociological issues see Therese A. Rando, *Grief, Dying, and Death: Clinical Interventions for Caregivers*, (Champaign, Illinois: Research Press Company, 1984), pp. 173–197.

6. It is noteworthy that Lindemann states that these techniques for grief reaction management "can be done in eight to ten interviews." I contend that this creates the impression that there is a standard amount of sessions/interviews needed to accomplish or in which one could accomplish management of grief reactions. This particular element of Lindemann's study appears to be at odds with my point that each person's uniqueness and special needs must be taken into consideration in order for the bereaved person to deal with death in a healthy fashion and in order for the caregiver to help the bereaved person manage his grief reactions. Lindemann was concerned with trying to break through the barrier of *not* attempting to assuage grief by psychiatric intervention. Thus, we should not focus on his time or session estimate but on the idea of addressing such needs in a timely, direct manner. Furthermore, we should strive to attain positive goals through therapy using a reasonable time frame in light of all important factors.

7. It is important to note that the main focus of self-help groups has undergone a shift in the past twenty years. For example, self-help groups such as Alcoholics Anonymous and Gamblers Anonymous have been based on the prohibitory philosophy of preventing people from doing something of a self-damaging and self-destructive nature in a proscriptive manner. Today, the central philosophy of the self-help groups is affirmatory and encourages members to do something for others as well as themselves.

8. There are numerous alternative skills appropriate in the education of health care professionals. The earlier cited recent publication on bereavement education contains suggestions that include "attentive listening . . . continuing the relationship with the bereaved . . . empathy with the bereaved . . . personal coping strategies . . . observational skills . . . and appropriate referrals." For a full discussion of their position see Osterweis, Solomon, and Green (eds.), *Bereavement: Reactions, Consequences, and Care, op. cit.*, pp. 215–236.

REFERENCES

Bowlby, J. 1969. *Attachment and Loss, Volume 1: Attachment.* New York: Basic Books, Inc.

Durkheim, E. 1915. *The Elementary Forms of Religious Life.* New York: The Free Press.

Firth, R. 1964. *Elements of Social Organization.* Boston: Beacon Press.

Freud, S. 1959. "Mourning and Melancholia." *Collected Papers.* New York: Basic Books, pp. 152–170.

Lindemann, E. 1944. "The Symptomatology and Management of Acute Grief." *American Journal of Psychiatry* 101:141–148.

Malinowski, B. 1948. *Magic, Science and Religion.* Garden City, New York: Doubleday and Co., Inc.

Osterweis, M., F. Solomon, and M. Green, eds., 1984. *Bereavement: Reactions, Consequences, and Care.* Washington, D.C.: National Academy Press.

Parkes, C.M. 1972. *Bereavement: Studies of Grief in Adult Life.* New York: International Universities Press, Inc.

Pine, V.R. 1972. "Social Organization and Death." *Omega* 3:149–153.

Rando, T.A. 1984. *Grief, Dying, and Death: Clinical Interventions for Caregivers.* Champaign, Illinois: Research Press Company.

30

THE EDUCATION OF PRECLINICAL MEDICAL STUDENTS IN THANATOLOGY

Frederick A. Ehlert

The education of medical students in thanatology is a highly relevant topic for study and discussion. In the past, experts have been assembled to present their analyses of the approaches to this area of medical education and have offered a broad spectrum of curriculum designs (Schoenberg et al. 1981). The focus of this chapter, however, is narrower and limited to the education of the preclinical medical student in thanatology.

The limited focus of this discussion results from two major concerns of mine. First, I am concerned over my own limitations. As a second year medical student, I am limited not only by time and space, but also by intellectual and professional experience. I have not yet experienced the clinical years of medical school, much less internship and residency. I do not really know what the third and fourth years of medical school involve. This limits my ability to understand how one learns to cope with death, loss, and grief in the role of clinician. This lack of experience may seem to restrict my ability to analyze the requirements and content of my own professional training. It need not be seen in such a light. Rather, it provides me with an advantage: I can observe the system from within. My second year standing allows me to report the observations, experiences, impressions, and feelings of a student in the midst of the "basic sciences" curriculum. The report is then a direct one, not tempered by time and not seen in the perspective of further educational trials.

My second concern is over the way the education of first and second year students in thanatology is viewed. The education of preclinical medical students is quite far removed from human issues in surgical care. In some sense the two are far apart. There is no need to convince this second year student how little he knows about anatomy, much less the surgical specialties. But, in thanatology, issues concerning both students and surgeons are interrelated. The first two years of medical school were for students of the past and remain for students of the present of vital importance in the development of professional character. For the first time in their lives, medical students in the first and second years see themselves as future physicians. For the first time, they are trying to act and react to stressful medical situations as they feel physicians should. Making this situation even more complex and more important is the fact that these students have, at the same time, limited experience in the medical world and limited exposure to professionals who can act as role models. Because of this, the impact of each experience is amplified and the impression each experience makes lasts longer than at any other time in medical education. By studying these "basic sciences" years, surgeons can reflect on their own education and the formation of their own attitudes and values. And, they can see the impact they have on first and second year students, not only in the formation of a preclinical data base, but also in the accumulation and formation of attitudes and values regarding death, dying, and bereavement.

To understand the education of first and second year medical students in thanatology we must first find where students encounter death and dying. What do we have available to teach students? Where do they learn to cope with death, dying, and bereavement? Some obvious answers to these questions present themselves. These answers are the parts of the "basic sciences" curriculum labeled thanatology in big, bold letters. First on this list are the courses that have been added to the curriculum in the past few years. These courses emphasize the interaction between physician and patient as more than simply diagnosis and treatment of disease. At the College of Physicians and Surgeons of Columbia University one such course, entitled *Introduction to the Practice of Medicine* (or ITTPM), covers topics including the physician-patient relationship, the interaction between society and medicine, and the health care system, as well as introducing students to many different medical specialties and teaching students how to conduct a physical exam. In this course, students have the opportunity to meet patients who have suffered loss—for example, alcoholics, insulin-dependent diabetics, paralyzed patients, and the elderly. These first interactions with patients are nurtured and the impact on both students and patients is discussed. This course meets for most of the first and second years, one afternoon per week.

Also included in this category of "obvious" thanatology are some sections and lectures of larger courses that are usually more oriented toward the basic sciences. These segments attempt to show students the relationship between the hard science and its impact on patients. The Abnormal Human Biology course, oncology section, devotes part of its syllabus and lecture time to "Physician-Patient Communication Patterns in the Clinical Setting; Implications for the Involvement of Medical Students with Cancer Patients." One of the lectures and a chapter of the course syllabus in Psychiatry is entitled "The Responsibilities of the Physician Towards the Dying Patient." Finally, and not to be forgotten, are electives for first and second year students. These electives are nine hours in length and scheduled during students' free time.

These courses are hardly the only places medical students encounter death and dying. Many other courses and many other experiences teach preclinical students how to cope with death, dying, and bereavement without the labels "thanatology" or "death and dying" attached to them. This way of learning about death arises from the very nature of medical school: students are required to learn the normal structure and function of the human body and the disease-states that alter those normals. These diseases imply suffering, they imply loss, and they imply death. Learning about them necessitates a response, a reaction by students, and a mechanism to cope with that reaction. The impact of these nonlabeled thanatology courses cannot be overemphasized; much more time is spent learning diseases than could ever be devoted officially to thanatology. Also, the influence of this type of learning is more subtle; it is not labeled, it is not brought to the attention of students or faculty, it might not even be brought to the attention of the conscience. Still it is present, in every lecture students attend, in every text students read. It is probably where students learn most how to deal with death, dying, and bereavement.

The not-so-obvious encounters that teach students how to cope might best be illustrated by examples. One example is the gross anatomy course. Gross anatomy laboratory is, for many students, the first time they see a dead body. The course requires that they not only see it, but that they dissect and study it. The manner in which this encounter is presented and developed by the faculty is extremely important in teaching acceptable and unacceptable coping mechanisms. In the first lecture both the course director and the associate course director told students:

> The cadaver was at one time a living, breathing, feeling human being. This person thought enough of medical science and of *your* education to give this ultimate gift. . . . This cadaver represents a significant financial investment on the part of the school and a significant human investment on the part of that person and his family. It is your responsibility to take care of it and respect it as such. . . .

That is a good encounter with thanatology and an appropriate framework in which to learn to cope with death. Not all encounters provide such guidance.

Another example of an encounter with thanatology in the first and second years is in the biochemistry course, where students learn the pathways, enzymes, and mechanisms the body uses to sustain life. Medical students must, of course, also learn about the cases when those enzymes do not work the way they were meant to. In biochemistry, these cases are termed "inborn errors of metabolism," a phrase students hear from almost the first lecture in the course. Often, this enzyme failure means the patient will die, or in biochemistry terminology the defect is "incompatible with life." In the clinical correlation part of the course, patients, usually babies, are presented to the class in a lecture hall, signs and symptoms are reviewed, and students see and hear just how "incompatible with life" the problem is. The patient is removed from the room, and the failed enzymes and pathways are discussed. This, too, educates medical students in death and dying; this, too, necessitates learning how to cope, but in this case the framework for coping presented to students is less desirable. It involves technological and intellectual isolation.

This leads to a second area that must be studied in order to understand thanatology education for preclinical medical students: the effectiveness of current efforts. There should be a comprehensive and scientific analysis of student attitudes toward thanatology and related topics looking for positive and negative changes that occur as a result of the preclinical years. While this type of study would probably be of great value to both faculty and students, the time and resources necessary would be immense. A large scale operation of this sort is not what I have in mind when I speak of evaluating effectiveness. A simpler and more immediately applicable way begins with a consciousness and awareness of *all* the messages that are being presented to students about thanatology. In other words, it is a self-analysis and self-critique undertaken by everyone involved in the education process, at every step of the education process. To assess the effectiveness, faculty and students, as joint participants in education, must ask themselves:

Are enough formal opportunities provided for education in thanatology?

How well are these presented?

Are all the informal opportunities that present themselves being used?

How well are these being used?

Do the formal and informal presentations complement one another? These are undoubtedly general questions, but their value lies not in the general answers or in the generalized discussion they may generate. The value is instead found in applying these questions to specific instances. Each lecture or part of a lecture, each potential encounter with death, loss or grief needs to be evaluated in this way.

Another example might best illustrate this point. One part of the anatomy course at CUP&S is correlation clinic, lectures in which surgeons relate the anatomy unit being studied to procedures, techniques, and approaches used in surgery. When the perineum is studied, one of the correlation clinics focuses on testicular cancer surgery and the techniques used in orchiectomy. In this lecture, the surgeon discussed how the approach is inguinal rather than transscrotal to limit lymphatic spread of malignant cells. He also discussed new combined chemotherapy treatments and new hormonal tests of treatment efficacy. While these techniques were being presented, all the male students in the lecture hall were squirming in their seats, many convinced they had testicular tumors and most imagining some degree of pain. The lecturer kept forging ahead with techniques and technology. Toward the end of the lecture, he covered the "obvious effects on the patient's self-image" along with the need for cosmetic restructuring and sperm-banking. But all the good things he had to say in the formal presentation of thanatology were lost because of all the things he avoided saying in the informal presentation. The effectiveness of his efforts was significantly diminished, not because of a lack of opportunities or awareness of thanatology, not because of inadequacies in his formal thanatology presentation, but because of a failure to use the right opportunities. And we missed an excellent opportunity to educate first and second year students in thanatology.

To understand thanatology education for preclinical medical students, we must also look at the other factors that influence the way students receive the messages that are being sent. There are many other encounters, completely unrelated to thanatology, that affect the way students respond to the programs and lectures designated thanatology. Understanding these other factors can make presentations, both formal and informal, more available and effective. In the first two years of medical school, three major forces influence students: administration, faculty, and fellow students. Each of these plays a role in the impact of education in thanatology on students. Each can contribute to or detract from the final message received by students.

Administration plays a large role in developing curriculum for the first and second years. It is one group responsible for increasing formal exposure of medical students to thanatology. This group thought enough of courses like ITTPM to add them to an already tight schedule, an addition which sends one message to students about the importance of the course. But students also receive conflicting messages from scheduling practices; when exam time roles around, the schedule, with all its additions from recent years, stops and exams start. The tests are in courses like anatomy, physiology, and pharmacology. The other courses fall to the wayside until tests are over. The message students get from this is clear: anatomy, physiology, pharmacology, and other "major" courses are important ones. If their schedule gets tight, students decide that these are the courses to attend and these are the texts to study. We must look also at the assignment of faculty to direct these courses. The people that run the "major" courses are usually senior faculty, often tenured professors, with long white coats and distinguished-looking silver hair. Courses with less basic science emphasis, including the courses containing most of the formal thanatology, are run by younger, junior faculty members with no power and probably no tenure. Again, the message students get from this is that the hard science courses are more important. Certainly, these courses are important; there is no question about that. The question that does arise in students' minds, however, is why are the thanatology courses in the curriculum? Did we add these courses simply to complete a list in the course catalogue, or did we do so out of a commitment to teaching students about subjects like thanatology?

Much of this paper alludes to the direct role faculty play in thanatology education. The indirect role must also be considered. How does the interaction between faculty and students in the overall basic science education affect thanatology education? One major consideration here is the emphasis placed on information presented in lectures and the manner in which that emphasis is applied. There is an incredible amount of material to be covered in every course, especially in basic science courses. Often so much material must be presented on a topic that it becomes hard for faculty to fit it all in the fifty minute time-slot allotted each lecture. But, too often and too easily the focus becomes solely that information and its presentation. Information is presented in lecture, studied by students, and tested with multiple choice questions and never once thought about. Alzheimer's Disease becomes *only* neurofibrillary tangles, senile plaques, and granulovascular degeneration rather than a disease with those morphologic alterations that causes immense suffering to patients and family—it is!—but so, too, are the human implications of that information. How often are medical students really confronted with those difficult implications by their teachers? When students are not confronted in lectures and discussions, when students are tested with only multiple choice questions, it becomes too easy for them to avoid the difficult, painful implications of disease and of death. Being allowed to avoid by the faculty makes avoidance easier.

Finally, we come to the role students play in all this. I must admit, as a student, this is the most difficult area to objectively and critically analyze. Some facts, though, are too obvious to miss. One is that students exert little effort in thanatology and related areas. This past November, the second year death and dying elective had one student sign up out of a class of 150. Granted, this was an elective taken during the one free afternoon scheduled per week, but this is hardly an acceptable percentage. Another obvious fact is that students have all sorts of excuses for not being interested or not taking time. Major blame is placed on the schedule ("we already spend too much time in class") and on the workload ("we already have all this material to know, how can I be expected to think about the impact?" or "why should I spend time on things I can't be tested on?") As a student I sympathize with these complaints. The schedule is full and there is a seemingly endless amount of material to know, but these demands do not decrease the importance of thanatology. Neither do these demands necessarily make students better equipped to handle issues of death, dying, and bereavement when these issues confront them as they eventually and inevitably will. Students must take some initiative for thanatology education to be taught them.

In summation, what I have tried to emphasize is the necessary commitment that thanatology education of preclinical medical students requires.

31

THE RESIDENT'S PERSPECTIVE

KARIN M. MURASZKO

W hat is the role of the resident with respect to interactions with attendings, medical students, family members, and patients?

Although a medical degree has been awarded, it does not invest its recipient with instantaneous insight or the ability to cope with the complex issues associated with a dying patient. As in most of medicine, time provides for assimilation of a multitude of experiences that then provide a basis from which an approach can be determined. The resident is a part of a continuum of education which begins with the medical student, inexperienced, naive and searching for role models, knowledge of what to do, how to do it and when to do it. It ends with the attending who is more knowledgeable about how to manage a variety of situations, though still puzzling on occasion about the wisdom of his decisions. The intervening years between medical school and actual medical practice are designed to provide the individual with a personally fashioned scheme for dealing with complex problems. Such a scheme not only acts to help a doctor efficiently handle a problem but also provides the necessary "knee jerks" and compulsiveness that permit the physician to obtain the maximum amount of information as smoothly and effectively as possible.

It is the purpose of residency programs to prepare an individual for the myriad of responsibilities that a physician must assume. The preparatory process places the individual in a unique set of circumstances, designed to train him to face being in a difficult position. The resident functions in a series of quasi-roles. Although he is no longer a medical student, by virtue of his inexperience, he may well still feel he is acting as a student, particularly at the beginning. Yet a transition is occurring whereby he is assuming more and more responsibility for patients and for the decisions he makes regarding those patients.

Medical students, particularly, are aware of the resident's position and role in the management team. Interviewed students have stated that because of the amount of time spent with the resident staff, they found them to be a significant if not the most significant part of their learning experience, particularly on the general surgery clerkship. Students identify with the resident and although they will also make use of the attending staff, they will frequently place the resident in the position of role model. This may well be the first time the resident is acting as a teacher and he may be unaware that he is, in fact, a role model for students.

The resident must successfully interact as well with various more senior members of the team, i.e., the attending staff. This is, in general, among the most difficult tasks that the resident must perform. He is responsible, on the one hand, for carrying out the wishes of the attending staff yet is, at the same time, developing his own independent style and methods for dealing with patients and their problems. It is in striking a balance that each resident generally finds he has the most difficult problems.

Realistically, the resident is often at the front lines where it comes to patient care and decision making. He is the one called into the patient's room for chest pain or abdominal discomfort. Yet he recognizes a sense of obligation to the attending physician; for the attending is ultimately responsible for the individual patient. The resident is acting as an ambassador for the attending. A balance between obligation and independence must be achieved, though at times this may be impossible.

The resident is aware that his actions will be under scrutiny from several levels. First and foremost, there is the patient, who in the hospitalization process has faced a variety of members of the medical community. Patients find it quite difficult to assign a role or level of importance to each member of the staff. Generally, they recognize their individual attending as the leader of the storm troopers in white. When it comes time to assign a role for the other members of the staff, patients will often assign levels of importance based on two aspects: First, who most effectively helped them with their day-to-day problems and needs; and second, who spent the greatest physical time with them, particularly time talking.

This can cause a skew in the natural order of things. Much to the medical student's surprise, he may take on a significance to the patient which supersedes that of the senior resident and, on occasion, even that of the attending.

The resident, in trying to deal effectively with the patient, is attempting to apply humane standards of care but also senses a pressure with respect to allocations of time. There is a sense of frustration because of the continuous conflict within and around him. He is attempting to be a competent and mature physician, but his authority is being challenged by the patient, the attending, and even the medical student. He is at the front lines but the decision-making process is often elsewhere. He is merely the bearer of the bad tidings: "I'm sorry Mrs. Jones, you need another IV." "Okay, Mrs. Jones, this will only hurt for a short time; your doctor ordered that we debride this wound." He wants to be kind to his patients but he is in a headlong risk to complete his various daily duties, please his attendings, spend hours in apprenticing in the craft of surgery, and trying to catch rare moments to read and learn a little more. Somewhere in a given day, it is just difficult to find enough time and draw forth from the depths of a fatigued and frustrated breast, the compassion that he would like to extend to a patient.

These issues are especially difficult where one is dealing with a critically ill or terminally ill patient. In situations such as those confronted in the intensive care unit or the emergency room, the resident staff is particularly pressured. Patients are seriously ill, situations change in a minute-by-minute fashion. At most institutions, such areas are almost entirely resident run. It is these areas of the hospital where residents are asked to make a large number of decisions quickly. There is frequently insufficient time to discuss all the medical problems and alternative plans, let alone appreciate the psychosocial implications of each decision. It is here, as well, that breakdown in communication occurs, particularly between the attending staff and residents. At times, the resident staff is with patients for longer periods of time than the attending staff. There may be a natural transference of increasingly larger amounts of responsibility to the resident, by both the patient and the staff. In many cases, however, the ultimate decision regarding life and death issues such as intubation, further therapy, repeated transfusions and ultimately termination of life support systems is made by a voice over the phone. Residents walk a difficult tight rope in that they wish to assume more responsibility yet may feel ill equipped to accept that responsibility for decisions. Residents state that the most effective management of patients has come from serious, open discussions with an involved attending, not some distant voice dispensing orders.

We are also cognizant of our mortality and our own frailty. In dealing with seriously ill patients on a daily basis, we must suppress these feelings to allow us to go on. Like most good students of introductory psychiatry, we are also aware that what we suppress will surface in the most unusual way. Each of us recognizes at some level that we are humans treating other humans and, as such, capable of being affected by the same terrible processes that are ravaging our patients. It would be ludicrous, however, to dwell on these issues for we would spend our time not healing or helping those who need our help but grieving about imaginary ills that might befall us.

Residents, particularly, develop a wall between themselves and their dying patients. It is evident in the jokes, the necessary euphemisms, and finally even by the simplest and most overlooked form of medical intervention, our conversations with patients. How does one handle the following situation? Mr. Jones has had a biopsy two days ago. The resident has in his possession the pathology report. He knows that there is a malignancy but also knows that the attending physician won't be in to see the patient until the next day. The patient is distraught and anxious to know the results of the biopsy. The solution for the resident is a simple one. He may either lie or he may simply choose to avoid the patient and his family. When next he makes his rounds, he will at best dart in and out of the room and utter reassuring platitudes with a deadpan face. What if the attending physician has informed the patient of his diagnosis? What can and can't the resident say to the patient? How much does the patient really know? The attending physician may have painted a picture of the situation different from that which the resident believes to be true. The resident finds himself asking the patient, "Well Mr. Jones, I'm sure you've had a talk with your attending. What exactly did Dr. X tell you?" He may simply not be certain about what the attending believes about a particular situation. Worse yet, he may philosophically disagree with the attending. What does one do then?

The job of a resident is sufficiently difficult that to consider all of the social ramifications of a particular decision may lead him to avoid the problem entirely. It becomes simpler, more efficient, less time consuming and certainly less likely to bring forth the wrath of an attending simply to avoid talking to the patient.

I know of no resident, particularly at the junior level, who has not told a patient—"I'm sorry, I have to run. I just don't have time to talk with you." Hours are long, personal time is short, and the workload enormous. As has been suggested by many attendings, the residency teaches one to cut corners. A quick way to do that is to not talk to your patients. "It doesn't affect their operation and has little affect on their care." Such statements demonstrate just how sorry the state of affairs can be for a surgical resident, and even more importantly for his or her patients. The patient is denied a complete team and must rely on the surgical attending for empathy and awareness.

In the midst of this conflict is the medical student, trying to find a role model and a direction. He senses, if not learns of, the conflict in opinions between resident and attending. He or she is not sure how to resolve the problems. He fears reprisal by either group, for his evaluation and grades depend on everyone "liking" him. What then does one do? Often the solution is to throw oneself into the science of the job, ignoring the humanity of it all as much as possible. Each case is a set of right answers, a chance to display knowledge. Avoid conflict, and get through to the next rotation.

The situation turns into one in which the attending may be giving a patient one particular party line, the resident another, and the medical student a third. One can only guess what the rest of the health care system and family might be saying. All participants in the process are trying to keep themselves functioning and the care of the patient is being fragmented. Family and friends must find this system even more difficult to cope with as the apparent hierarchy and significance of each individual on the team blurs.

I'm not sure that I can offer specific solutions to these problems. They demonstrate that we at times fail to effectively care for our patients. Yes, we provide them with medical care but we often fail to provide them with total care. It is an impossible task to simply say "make it better." The key seems to be to open up the channels of communication. Sometimes the solutions come from the most unlikely places. If the team members were capable of communicating with each other, there would be a more effective, cohesive, and perhaps even compassionate group offering aid to the patient.

Among the most effective working situations I have experienced was one in which an attending at some point during the day, simply paged me or pulled me aside and spent 10 minutes reviewing his patients and their specific problems, medical or otherwise. I believe this actually saved time and in the end helped open up further avenues of communication. I think these patients received better care and all involved with them felt more relaxed. The team was working as a team and had a game plan, a unified care plan for each patient with a strong leader guiding that plan. With increasing experience the resident assumes more of this responsibility and becomes himself such a leader for those patients under his direct and total care.

There is no pat solution for these complex issues. Further, it is the purpose of this discussion to prompt introspective analysis of the nature of the interaction within the caregiving team, particularly the relationship between the resident and the attending physician. So much of what we accomplish with patients is accomplished not with the knife but with the word and the touch. It is unfortunate that we do not use these techniques not just to heal our patients but to heal ourselves. We are part of a community which has elected to spend its life caring for the injured and sick among us. Nowhere is that care more needed than in the critically and terminally ill patient for whom there are no simple answers and for whom this may be their final time. We must be mindful of the very definition of the word community and remember that without the ability to commune, there can be no unified patient care.

We do ourselves, our profession, our students and most importantly our patients a serious disservice if we fail to be open for discussion, to be able to display our humanity. For John Donne was correct, "Everyman is a piece of the Continent, a part of the main." We need to be open and complete in our discussions about life and death, pain and treatment, options and inevitabilities. We all hope that discussions are available for us when we no longer are a member of the caregiving team but the object of its care.

32

EDUCATION IN THANATOLOGY—
THE PRACTITIONER

MILTON W. HAMOLSKY

Historically—and in broad, general terms—the practitioner (here defined as the physician—surgeon, internist, family practitioner) has emerged progressively in this country from the turn of the century as the prime advocate and decision maker for his/her individual patient and family unit. The "good ole family doctor" of fond nostalgia delivered babies, managed colic or Colles fractures, observed congenital heart disease and rheumatic fever, shared as confidant and counselor in the growth and development of the individual and the family to adulthood and old age, managed trauma and heart attacks and strokes and family crises, shared also—with empathy and dignity but without much other effective therapy—the at home, bedside dying of meningitis or influenza or cancer; and he accepted, with variable equanimity, his pedestalled position, and shared with patients the dominant inevitability of death—virtually an act of God—dwarfing his limited diagnostic and therapeutic armamentaria. Because of this gross and real disproportion, the realistic expectations of both patients and practitioners were low. Societal respect and reverence and dependence grew, based on evidences that the doctor "did the very best he could," that his was the best authority on prognosis, that he knew best and dispensed the currently available therapies, unchallenged by prospective, double-blind, crossover studies, unfettered by morbidity and mortality and quality-assurance reviews.

One other theme of this prologue to counterpoint merits consideration. Around the turn of the century, over 90 percent of people died at home, stereotypically the center of the entire family's participatory attention and sharing dedication. Although current home-care programs and the growing emergence of the hospice concepts have rediscovered the putative values of dealing with dying at home, the institutionalization of dying remains dominant, attributed to diverse social, economic, technologic, and psychologic forces. Today's practitioners and aspirants to the profession, therefore, have missed the entrainment upon their DNA or RNA—or hypothalamus—of this profound intellectual and emotional experience. Each year, I ask the entering freshmen of Brown's Program in Medical Education how many had personally experienced the dying of a parent or grandparent or sibling in the home situation; each year less than 1 percent respond positively.

Major advances in public health and the prevention of bacterial diseases, in the individual and epidemically, followed by the endless proliferation and striking effectiveness of antibiotics have diminished both the reality and the resigned acceptance of the lethal scourge of infections—diphtheria, meningitis, tuberculosis, bacterial endocarditis, and the old man's friend, pneumonia. "God's will" has become "medicine's failure," increasing society's expectations, the practitioner's responsibility, and human longevity—effecting the emergence of the chronic, disabling, complex, and costly diseases of the proliferating elderly.

Unimagined advances in basic scientific knowledge—qualitatively, quantitatively, and in explosive profusion and speed from the laboratory to the bedside—have provided the practitioner with the potential for *and* the challenge of a more scientifically precise base for diagnosis, therapy, and prognosis. The generalist has been overwhelmed by information overload, contributing to the rapid growth of specialization with its resultant fragmentation of health care, leading inexorably to the increasing emergence of the clichéd multidisciplinary approach—forcing the once vaunted, all-knowing professor to become increasingly the conductor of the medical care symphony and the practitioner, hopefully, the quarterback and coach and general manager of the medical team.

Similarly, the identification, isolation, purification, synthesis, and chemical manipulation of a profusion of chemical agents—with increasing knowledge of mechanisms of biosynthesis, secretion, transport, receptor binding and ultimate biological effects—of vitamins, hormones, enzymes, anesthetic agents, tranquilizers, analogues, agonists, antagonists—have provided the practitioner with unimagined power for pharmacologic good for patients—and potential for harm.

When I was an intern, a patient who suffered a heart attack received 5–6 weeks of bed rest, oxygen, morphine, digitalis, quinidine, mercurial diuretics and, with variable degrees of certainty, anticoagulants, and survived—or, as often, died. Today's practitioner must encompass risk factor recognition, management, and optimistic prevention, precise invasive and noninvasive diagnostic technology, the decision to carry out—or postpone—bypass surgery, educated public cardiopulmonary resuscitation, municipal rescue teams, coronary care units with the skilled internist and nurse-specialist, monitors, pacemakers, respirators, balloon pumps, coronary angioplasty, coronary catheterizations, thrombolytic agents, calcium blockers, beta-blockers, an endless array of antiarrhythmics, inotropics, preload and afterload reducers—all compressed hectically within a 7- to 14-day acute phase leading promptly to the organized optimism of rehabilitation.

When I was an intern, patients with localized cancer might benefit from surgery or receive palliative radiation—and then die. Our current practitioners must deal positively—with a more knowledgeable and, thus, more expectant public—with prevention and early recognition, appropriate staging (with CAT scanners, invasive and digital angiography, radioactive scanning, and, just ahead, nuclear magnetic resonance) with Hobson's choices among advanced surgery, radiation therapy, the two-edged sword of chemotherapy, the ever-emerging new and hopeful experimental promise. Today's residents deal with patients with serious side effects, damaged bone marrows, depressed immune capacity, life-threatening susceptibility to infections and bleeding—a heartening increased survival potential, and the too ofter depressing recurrence.

It is precisely such advances in, and ultimate limitations of, the science and technology of biology and medicine that pose the awesome challenges and responsibilities to the practitioner's art of medicine. It is the control of infectious diseases, advances in neonatology, surgery for congenital diseases, antibiotics, chemotherapy, the pacemaker, the respirator, the SMA-20 battery of laboratory tests, the catheter, the fiberoptiscope, the promise, filled and unfulfilled, of research that have created the half-way technologies, have prolonged living, have permitted the artificial maintenance of biological survival. It is the contributions of philosophers, ethicists, sociologists, economists, psychologists, legislators, writers, lawyers, judges, hospital administrators, health-care planners and third-party payors that have added the unresolved and controversial dimensions of informed consent, of the newly articulated rights of the patient and the family to share in—or make—the definitive decision, of ethical, legal, and human issues involved in initiating and sustaining extraordinary measures of care, do-not-resuscitate orders, high cost transplantation, cost-effective analysis, defensive medicine in the face of an increasingly litigious society and escalating malpractice premiums, the "living will," the legal definition of death, a presidential commission, utilization reviews, PSRO's, the looming DRG reimbursement system—all highlighting starkly the practitioner caught between the conflicting pressure of his professional responsibility to his patient versus his societal responsibility to his greater community.

Nowhere is the resultant challenge to his art of medicine greater than in sharing the dying, death, and bereavement of his patient and the family.

What are the relevant requirements for the good practitioner? First is the solid base of scientific knowledge, tempered by clinical experience. Compassion and empathy alone will not suffice, even for his dying patient, if the physician has not mastered the skillful history, physical examination, judicious selection and critical interpretation of diagnostic tests, and the slowly acquired skills of clinical synthesis and judgment—if he misses the changing heart murmur, the unequal pupils, the drug-induced somnolence or agitation, the depression due to hypothyroidism. The realistic acceptance of the incurable state does not terminate this basic obligation of the professional. More difficult usually, and therefore more demanding, is the professional maturation and inner security to avoid yet another x-ray, another battery of lab tests, another round of chemotherapy—but just to sit and listen unhurriedly, to alleviate with equal concentration insomnia, anorexia, constipation, pain, to enlist the special contributions of nurses, social workers, religious advisors, but sustain for the long haul his central role, refusing the tempting diversion of the unpleasant to others. He must—in sum—balance in varying degrees at different junctures the roles of the critical scientist, the skilled clinician, and the humanistic "good ole family doc."

I mentioned above our personal and collective experiential poverty in regard to dying and death. Thus deprived, our practitioner-to-be is caught up in our youth-oriented society, which extols the virtues of action, of virility, of athletic prowess, denigrating by avoidance the process of aging and by denial, the inevitability of death. Reinforcement of attitude and denial of a value or meaning for dying are nurtured during four years of medical school's primacy of scientific knowledge, clinical diagnosis, technical virtuosity in treatment and cure—or, occasionally admitted, only significant alleviation of suffering of the depersonalized stroke or cancer or heart attack. Thus misled, our fresh and eager intern is shaken by the perverse persistence of chronic and incurable disease of the elderly, discouraged by the repetitious return, in November, of the little old lady he rejuvenated in August, and shocked by death despite his—and medicine's—best efforts. For in his context, death is failure—and failure is handled by avoidance, by the brief, hurried visit, the superficial question without time for an answer and—at the end, the formalized pronouncement of death, request for an autopsy, and abandonment of the body to the nurse.

But this selectively bleak and extreme scenario is changing, sometimes slowly, but inexorably gathering momentum. And I can conclude with a heartening kaleidoscope of some of the emerging forces that serve as tribute to our good practitioner of the present and as guideposts for our good practitioner of the future.

We now share in a society that has been sensitized and shaken by the civil rights movement, the Vietnam War, the triumph of the scientific mind in probing the secrets of the atom and the overbalancing threat of nuclear war, the horrors of the holocaust, the feminist movement and the leavening increase of women in medicine, the landing of man on the moon and space shuttles, the dialysis machine and the artificial heart, therapeutic abortion and test-tube babies, the awesome computer and the invasion of privacy, the instant display and replay of history by the relentless television tube, capital punishment and white collar crime, Karen Quinlan and Baby Doe. I sense that our young men and women of medicine today are more aware of the world around them, more sensitive to the rights of others, more caring, more involved than I and my colleagues were but a few years ago at a comparable stage of development.

Troubled by a growing discomfort and dissatisfaction with the medical education process at both national and local levels, leaders and shapers have launched a vigorous attack on the curriculum, eschewing the ubiquitous 5–7 year cosmetic reshuffling. The essentials of the core curriculum are under debate and redefinition. The infantilization of the university graduate in medical school by repetitive lectures, merciless stuffing with evanescent esoterica and memorized regurgitation is yielding, reluctantly, to a hoped-for, intellectual excitement and challenging commitment to become the perpetual self-learner. We are incorporating, more honestly, the continuum of the long respected but neglected humanities, the arts and literature, sociology, anthropology, psychology and psychiatry, population and family interactions, economics, ethics, communication skills, psychosocial sensitivities.

The subjects of death and dying have been both subjected to extensive study by the humanists and ethicists and popularized in the media. More and more schools of medicine now engage their students in serious considerations of these issues—at both the personal and societal levels.

The resurgence of family practice, general internal medicine, primary care, required longitudinal immersion in outpatient and ambulatory experience with emphasis on sustained continuity are gradually elevating the personal fulfillments and satisfactions of dedicated care of the common headache, backache, shifting aches and pains, adolescent turbulence, reactive depression, and the dying patient as counterpoint to the "interesting" disseminated lupus erythematosis and ectopic ACTH production.

More and more residency training programs now grapple openly with such problems in discussion groups permitting shared verbalizations of individual culture shocks of sudden responsibilities for sick human beings, unremitting stress and fatigue, disappointments and frustrations. Our residents are now exposed to ethics committees, to patients' rights, society's pleas for some limitations of extraordinary methods reflexly sustained. Our good practitioner, therefore, has been sensitized, has achieved a measure of self-recognition and personal resolution of his own mortality, and recognizes such problems more readily in his dying patient and tries to help his patient to acknowledge, to verbalize, to understand, to suffer, to mourn, to accept, to adjust, to achieve some comfort in open sharing with the doctor and associates, with family and friends. He strives to understand the prior capacities and individualities of his patients, to estimate the overall quality and meaning of the living which accompanies his efforts, share the pros and cons with involved family members, and devise an appropriate and measured therapeutic and selective diagnostic management, ready and secure to discontinue extraordinary measures within the context of each patient and family unit.

He eschews the misleading circumlocution, he insists on honesty and integrity of communication but with patience, a slow and measured unfolding of the medical truths, attuned to the tolerance of his patient. He knows of the terrible loneliness of the dying patient, of the fear of rejection and he persists in multiple visits, always impressing with an unhurried and patient-focused visit (even if time pressures limit the actual stay), intuitively judging the appropriateness of a light and bantering interchange, or a serious, even solemn discussion probing the depths of feeling because it is wanted and needed, or just holding the hand without unnecessary or irrelevant words. He can accept, and adjust to, the unorthodox and self-directed therapies of a Norman Cousins. He warms the stethoscope diaphragm before placing it against the chest. He somehow manages to be there when his patient is on a narrow, hard stretcher on the way to the unknown of the operating room or the cardiac catheterization. He anticipates the deep fears of pain, or disfigurement, or incapacity and dependence on others, of financial drain to loved ones and he guarantees at least relief from pain and a caring concern and realistic commitment to share in facing the other problems. He educates the family about the patient's fear of abandonment so they can face the patient more honestly and share the experience for whatever mutual strengths may eventuate. He knows about the principles and services of the hospice programs and effects their participation when appropriate. He explores the religious background of his patient and its importance and engages the help of the priest or rabbi. He seeks help from social service and continues to share in their efforts, rather than assuaging himself that "they" will take off those "kind of problems." He discusses the relevant issues with the nurses, participates obviously with them and the patient in joint evaluation of responses to therapy and planning for the next steps. He appreciates the trauma of the unknown and strives to report promptly the results—and meaning—of yesterday's tests and discuss informatively the next day's procedures that are planned. He engages the patient as a partner in a joint effort rather than the unknowing recipient of his orders. He inquires about appetite, the food, sleep, bowel habits, the grandchildren, reading, sports, hobbies, and he always remembers to ask, "Do you understand? Is that clear? Do you have any questions?"— and he waits for the answers.

And he perseveres—equally in the face of "good news" and a grateful patient or "bad news" and a dissatisfied or complaining or demanding patient and family and the ultimate challenge of dying—to alleviate pain and anxiety and fear, to extract dignity and meaning for this last phase of living, to share with compassion and gentle honesty and caring objectivity.

And our good practitioner continues to expose himself to educational programs that symbolize the growing body of knowledge and theory forged by students and teachers of the human and ethical issues involved in the totality of caring for the patient—as vital to his professional efforts as his proud heritage of science and technology. For—as stated and restated—"The secret of caring for the patient is indeed to care for the patient."

33

EDUCATION IN THANATOLOGY
FOR SOCIAL WORKERS

ABRAHAM LURIE

Education in thanatology involves many facets. It includes the practical application of knowledge of death and dying to relationship with patients and to their families. It involves becoming familiar with the literature on death, dying, anticipatory grief, and bereavement. But above all there is an educational need to help professionals come to terms with their own feelings about separation, loss, and death.

Fear of death is universal and adults, children, and professionals often experience feelings of anxiety, guilt, and abandonment when confronted with separation as a result of death and dying. While professionals may have cognitive understanding of the significance of death, nevertheless their own psychological coping patterns as they relate to this process can vary from professional to professional.

Unfortunately, not all of the efforts of professionals result in helping patients and their families come to terms with feelings about the loss of a loved one. We need to be able to live with some problems that are not intractable and yet learn how to benefit from such experiences. The following is a case example:

The effect of surgery and death on the L family was one of decompensation and total breakdown of family system. The patient was a 5-year-old white female admitted to hospital complaining of severe headaches, fever, and gastroenterology distress. Parents were first cousins, traditional, culturally old-world European. The extended family is very

227

close, and large numbers of relatives were always at the hospital. The parents had another 3-year-old daughter, but had lost one child in infancy prior to the patient's birth. They were strongly religious and accepted deaths as God's will. The patient's bed was surrounded with pictures of religious symbols.

The patient was in intensive care unit seven months, during which brain surgery was performed for placement of a shunt. Several exploratory intestinal surgeries were performed in a medical effort to locate the source of the patient's illness. Every branch of medicine was consulted as the patient continued to deteriorate. She eventually went into a coma, body systems began to shut down, and the patient was maintained on life supports.

The parents were initially supportive and appeared devoted to each other. Their lives totally revolved around the children and family. The father was very protective of the mother, sought to spare her pain, and occasionally withheld medical information. He was verbal, receptive to social work intervention, and had great faith in God and doctors. The mother tended to be more private, was not a good communicator, also had great faith in religion, and responded only to her priest. As patient's condition worsened, the mother became more withdrawn, refused nourishment, and rejected sleep. Her physical condition deteriorated, she had bouts of confusion, fainting episodes, and became a management problem for family and staff. She fluctuated between hysteria and despair, and the family feared she was a suicide threat. The pressure on the spouse was great, and he was unable to cope or understand his wife's behavior. He had his wife involuntarily committed to a psychiatric hospital. She was so angered at this that she refused to speak to him or any family member.

During the period of the mother's confinement, the patient died — still with an undiagnosed condition. The mother rejected the autopsy, stating "they've cut her enough." She would not allow religious burial, and reluctantly allowed only immediate family members to attend. When the mother was discharged from the hospital (3-week hospitalization), she refused to speak to her spouse, family, or priest. She made daily visits to the patient's grave, spent the rest of the time in bed. She moved into the patient's room at home. She provided only limited care for her other child and has not resumed other household chores. She has completely rejected religion. The father is in despair, confused, and hurt. He is experiencing tremendous feelings of guilt, loss, and rejection and has had to assume the caretaking role in the house.

Contact by the social worker has been through phone with this family, and it is more than two years since the patient's death. The parents' relationship has been severely damaged. The wife has limited communication with spouse, and is hostile to him. She has resumed care of her other child, but is disinterested and withdrawn.

The parents have rejected all psychological help. Father also has turned to his family for support.

It is interesting to note that the father can only recall a vision of the patient all swathed in bandages with tubes. During her surgery, he was devastated by her appearance and brought in pictures for all to see how beautiful she was, what lovely hair she had. They agonized over the mutilation to her body, her hairlessness, her suture lines. In the end, the surgery had been fruitless and the patient died of an unknown infection that was the source of her original complaint.*

Despite the fact that psychiatry, social work, and nursing seemed to be of little avail to deal with the after-effects of the patient's death, we have learned from the experience.

The special emphasis of the social worker which helps the family deal with this phenomenon requires an educational process that includes stress reduction. Social workers need to involve natural supports that can help to relieve some of the emotional stresses. A major problem that social workers face as they become involved in thanatological processes is that they may attempt to take too much on their own, overextending themselves. As a result, they experience a sense of burnout or have difficulty in coping.

The phenomenon of burnout is not unique to those who are working with death and dying. However, there is a special sense of burnout with the care of the terminal patient. Professionals reflect specific feelings when patients are dying or die, such as powerlessness, guilt, confusion, and alienation. Wanting a patient to live or die mirrors the bereaved person's feeling toward the deceased and very often the professionals as well. Sometimes health professionals resent the situation that they are in.

How to deal with this represents a major administrative and professional problem. One way might be to rotate staff after a period of time so

*The author acknowledges the efforts of Joyce Kates, social worker at Long Island Jewish-Hillside Medical Center, in the preparation of this case report.

that they may be exposed to additional areas that would provide new interest and motivation. Some may not desire any rotation and may feel that the experience with dying, anticipatory grief, and bereavement offers more than adequate opportunities for learning and growth which will enable them to remain in such work and make of it the kind of professional career that is of interest.

Another area is to develop some newer approaches and psychosocial intervention. One such technique which would arouse interest and perhaps be of help is role playing. Another is family therapy involving families as a group in discussions and discussing feelings related to death and dying.

Strategies to avert feelings of health professionals include the importance of having mutual supports at work and at home. At work, this involves group support and sharing of some of the feelings with peers and involved persons of other disciplines such as physicians, nurses, clerks. Cognitive clarification allows the professional to distinguish between what is real and what isn't. This legitimizes feelings and overreactions spurred on by those who are grieving. This can be accomplished with continuing education, varying work routines, staff development around issues of death and dying, and a group of practitioners around issues of stress. At home, health professionals should try to detach the work from home life, and involve themselves in hobbies, use of humor as well as limiting the emotional investment. These strategies should help to soften some of the strong feelings that are attendant to the process of thanatology.

The care of the dying often ignores natural support systems of families and friends. Professionals should not expect family members to be passive bystanders because this may make them feel useless, inadequate, and helpless. Social workers need to be taught ways of encouraging this natural support in care of the dying since it can make families helpful and reduce their stress and facilitate bereavement.

For families at risk, who take care of the dying, are increasingly vulnerable when psychic, social, and financial resources are depleted. Social workers need to be taught how to develop outreach programs which would create a continuity of care process. Availability and access to these services should be the task of the professional in charge and how social workers can make this happen should be part of the educational process in thanatology. Techniques such as role playing with family members is a particularly effective method of providing instruction. The development of networks that help to create "social aftercare" for families at risk should also be explored as a technique in education.

Social work education is under review for several reasons, including the demands upon the schools of social work by many of the health and welfare agencies whose programs are constantly changing to meet the needs of the various target populations with whom they are involved. The demand for specialized areas of competence has put a great strain on the curricula of the schools, particularly since the length of study in graduate schools is only two years. There has been considerable emphasis on including course content pertaining to the aged, health, and to some extent, thanatology, which is not surprising since all this content is interrelated.

There needs to be several cautions. It has been noted that interest in some of this content is transitory and may even be said to be "trendy." One strong recommendation would be for content concerning those areas that are needed for practice to be included as part of continuing staff development and educational programs in health care agencies. Courses, seminars, special lecturers, and conferences should be introduced into staff continuing education programs.

It behooves all professionals who are concerned about the effects of death and dying on staff to develop innovative educational approaches that include ventilation of feelings, new knowledge, and interpersonal dynamics to develop staff competence necessary to deal with this profound experience.

AUTHOR INDEX

233

SUBJECT INDEX

237